Psychotherapy for Immigrant Youth

Sita G. Patel • Daryn Reicherter
Editors

Psychotherapy for Immigrant Youth

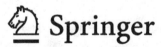 Springer

Editors
Sita G. Patel, PhD
Palo Alto University
Palo Alto, CA, USA

Daryn Reicherter, MD
Stanford University School of Medicine
Palo Alto, CA, USA

ISBN 978-3-319-24691-8   ISBN 978-3-319-24693-2   (eBook)
DOI 10.1007/978-3-319-24693-2

Library of Congress Control Number: 2015955252

Springer Cham Heidelberg New York Dordrecht London

Printed on acid-free paper

Springer International Publishing AG Switzerland is part of Springer Science+Business Media (www.springer.com)

I dedicate my work on this book to the members of my family. Their movements to and from all corners the globe reflect struggles and triumphs that fuel my passion for understanding and improving the lives of immigrant youth: Shardaben, Raojibhai, Leena, Ila, Arvind, Makrund, Aparna, Carol, Kiran, Shannon, Assefa, Doree, Julie, Jessica, Neeshan, Olivier, Hussein, Beletu, Mulumebet, Tewodros, Temesgen, and especially my wonderful husband, David.
—Dr. Patel

I, too, dedicate my work on this book to the members of my family. To my grandparents, Gerrit and Grace Dykstra and to my mother for showing courage and hope in their immigration to the United States. And I dedicate my work to my family: Ethan and Amelia, and especially my loving wife, Heidi.
—Dr. Reicherter

Introduction

Immigrant children and adolescents face many complex stressors—they must leave familiar people and routines, adjust to new social and academic norms, and navigate intersecting cultures. Although migration is rapidly increasing worldwide, and the risks to psychological health are clear, we know relatively little about best practices for conducting psychotherapy with immigrant youth. *Psychotherapy for Immigrant Youth* is an effort to advance the treatment of problems while building capacity and fostering resilience. This book describes the complex life experiences and psychological symptoms experienced by immigrant youth and takes an ecological-contextual approach to providing treatment. Symptoms and treatment delivery are intertwined with setting, and this book considers medical, community, and school environments, as well as the global contexts of receiving countries and low-resource settings. This book also addresses the complex and interconnected services required by immigrant families and their children, including housing and relocation, legal, and medication, and the ways that providers of psychotherapy can integrate these needs with their own services.

Psychotherapy for Immigrant Youth is intended for practitioners, researchers, and students who study and work with immigrant children and adolescents across multiple settings. Professionals in the fields of psychiatry, psychology, social work, public health, global mental health, and education will benefit from the book's practical and interdisciplinary approach. Each chapter provides an overview of related empirical work, applies a critical lens to the limitations of current knowledge, and provides suggestions for future directions and detailed case examples to illustrate issues and therapeutic techniques.

This book is a collection of chapters ordered into four parts that address themes essential to understanding different aspects of providing psychotherapy for immigrant youth.

The first part includes an analysis of the psychosocial stressors faced by immigrant youth. The chapter *Immigrant Youth Life Stressors* (Anna Staudenmeyer, Erynn Macciomei, Margareth Del Cid, and Sita G. Patel) introduces the complex life stressors faced by immigrant youth across the trajectory of pre-migration, through migration, and after settlement. This chapter clarifies the niche of psychotherapy for immigrant youth by contextualizing the special circumstances of cross-cultural mental health and social/legal circumstances faced by the population.

The second part provides a comprehensive review and concise discussion of contemporary, evidence-based psychotherapies for immigrant youth. Each chapter within this section highlights a specific treatment modality. The chapter *Cognitive-Behavioral Therapy for Immigrant Youth: The Essentials* (Micaela A. Thordarson, Marisa Keller, Paul J. Sullivan, Sandra Trafalis, and Robert D. Friedberg) provides an overview of core principles and techniques of cognitive behavior therapy, as they relate to immigrant youth. The chapter *Family Factors: Immigrant Families and Intergenerational Considerations* (Maryam Kia-Keating, Diana Capous, Linda Juang, and Guadalupe Bacio) focuses on the family, including family-level stressors and sources of resiliency. The chapter *School-Based Interventions* (Alisa B. Miller, Colleen B. Bixby, and B. Heidi Ellis) provides a review of the literature on school-based interventions with specific attention to comprehensive services for immigrant youth. It includes case examples of programs with good outcomes and effective interventions. The chapter *Trauma and Acculturative Stress* (John P. Rettger, Hilit Kletter, and Victor Carrion) first distinguishes between chronic stressors and acute trauma, then discusses frequent traumatic experiences faced by immigrant youth, and reviews current evidence-based treatment approaches for traumatized immigrant youth.

The third part of the book explores interventions and treatment modalities that are complementary to psychotherapy for immigrant youth. The chapter *Combined Psychotherapy with Psychopharmacology* (Yasmin Owusu) discusses challenges and considerations for the provision of psychiatric medication, including cultural and familial factors. The chapter *Information Systems and Technology* (Eduardo Bunge, Megan K. Jones, Benjamin Dickter, Rosaura Perales, and Andrea Spear) presents current practices related to integrating technology into psychotherapy.

The fourth and final part provides a discussion of using psychotherapy for immigrant youth within unique settings and some of the contextual challenges that may arise. The chapter *Treating Forcibly Displaced Young People: Global Challenges in Mental Healthcare* (Ruth V. Reed, Rebecca Tyrer, and Mina Fazel) highlights key features and challenges of various service delivery models in both low- and high-income settings and considers how resource differences influence the provision and sustainability of treatments with this heterogeneous population. The chapter *Immigrant Youth and Navigating Unique Systems That Interact with Treatment*, etc. (David E. Reed II, Marilee Ruebsamen, James Livingston, and Fazia Eltareb) explains the multiple, complex social systems that immigrant youth often require services for, including legal, medical, and educational. The book closes with the chapter *Cultural Perspectives in the Context of Western Psychological Mind-sets: The Need for Cultural Sensitivity in the Mental Health of Immigrant Youth* (Rania Awaad and Daryn Reicherter), which functions as a critical commentary on the challenges and limits of the applicability of Western brands of psychotherapy for non-Western individuals.

Psychotherapy for Immigrant Youth can be useful to practitioners section by section, chapter by chapter, or as a whole. The editors intended to create a volume that would inform and update the evidence base and also spark inquiry toward the questions and challenges that remain. Each section binds together several specific ideas into a theme, and each chapter is a stand-alone review with original and informative new ideas. The book, in total, intends to both inform and challenge the science and art of mental health practice for this vulnerable population.

May 2016   Sita G. Patel
                                                                                              Daryn Reicherter

The original version of this book was revised. An erratum to this book can be found at DOI 10.1007/978-3-319-24693-2_10

About the Editors

Sita G. Patel, Ph.D. is an Assistant Professor of Psychology at Palo Alto University. She is the director of the Cultural Transitions Research group and involved in Palo Alto University's programs for Global Mental Health, Trauma, and Diversity and Community Mental Health. She received a doctorate in clinical psychology from the University of California, Berkeley, with an emphasis on cultural and community psychology. She completed two years of postdoctoral training in community action research at the University of California, San Francisco. Dr. Patel's primary focus is on understanding the complex and interacting stressors facing newcomer immigrant adolescents, in particular among unaccompanied minors, as well as the clinical treatment of refugees from around the world. She also works with research teams in the Central African Republic and Kenya on projects aimed to reduce trauma, build peace, and strengthen community mental health. Dr. Patel's work involves multiple community partnerships with schools and clinics serving immigrant youth, and she is committed to fostering interdisciplinary team efforts.

Daryn Reicherter, M.D. is a Clinical Associate Professor of Psychiatry at Stanford University. He is director of the Human Rights in Trauma Mental Health Laboratory at Stanford. He is on the Fulbright Specialists roster for work in global trauma mental health. After receiving degrees in Psychobiology and Philosophy from the University of California at Santa Cruz, Dr. Reicherter completed his doctorate in medicine at New York Medical College. He completed internship and residency and served as Chief Resident at Stanford University Hospitals and Clinics. He is dedicated to providing a combination of administrative and clinical services in the area of cross-cultural trauma mental health. He works locally with refugee survivors from around the world. Dr. Reicherter is involved with the movement for promotion of trauma mental health and human rights issues spanning countries including Cambodia, Haiti, Zimbabwe, and Indonesia. He has published articles, chapters, and books on the topic of cross-cultural trauma. He has ongoing involvement in the advocacy for human rights in the area of war crime through the programs he serves, and beyond.

Contents

**Part IV   Special Circumstances for Psychotherapy
           for Immigrant Youth**

Contributors

Rania Awaad, M.D. Department of Psychiatry and Behavioral Sciences, Stanford Hospital, Stanford, CA, USA

Guadalupe Bacio, Ph.D. Department of Psychiatry, University of California, San Diego, San Diego, CA, USA

Eduardo Bunge, Ph.D. Palo Alto University, Palo Alto, CA, USA

Colleen B. Bixby, MPH Department of Psychiatry, Boston Children's Hospital, Boston, MA, USA

Victor Carrion, M.D. Stanford Early Life Stress & Pediatric Anxiety Program, Stanford, CA, USA

Diana Capous, M.A. Department of Counseling, Clinical and School Psychology, University of California, Santa Barbara, Santa Barbara, CA, USA

Margareth Del Cid, M.A. Pacific Graduate School of Psychology, Palo Alto University, Palo Alto, CA, USA

Benjamin Dickter, M.A. Palo Alto University, Palo Alto, CA, USA

B. Heidi Ellis, Ph.D. Department of Psychiatry, Harvard Medical School, Boston Children's Hospital, Boston, MA, USA

Fazia Eltareb, M.S. Palo Alto University, Palo Alto, CA, USA

Mina Fazel, M.R.C.Psych., D.M. Department of Psychiatry, University of Oxford, Warneford Hospital, Oxford, UK

Robert D. Friedberg Center for the Study and Treatment of Anxious Youth at Palo Alto University, Palo Alto University, Palo Alto, CA, USA

Megan K. Jones, B.S. Palo Alto University, Palo Alto, CA, USA

Linda Juang, Ph.D. Department of Education, Universität Potsdam, Potsdam, Germany

Marisa Keller, M.S. Center for the Study and Treatment of Anxious Youth at Palo Alto University, Palo Alto University, Palo Alto, CA, USA

Maryam Kia-Keating, Ph.D. Department of Counseling, Clinical and School Psychology, Gevirtz Graduate School of Education, University of California, Santa Barbara, Santa Barbara, CA, USA

Hilit Kletter, Ph.D. Stanford Early Life Stress & Pediatric Anxiety Program, Stanford, CA, USA

James Livingston, Ph.D. Asian Americans for Community Involvement, Center for Survivors of Torture, San Jose, CA, USA

Erynn Macciomei, M.S. Pacific Graduate School of Psychology, Palo Alto University, Palo Alto, CA, USA

Alisa B. Miller, Ph.D. Department of Psychiatry, Boston Children's Hospital, Harvard Medical School, Boston, MA, USA

Yasmin Owusu, M.D. Department of Psychiatry and Behavioral Sciences, Stanford Hospital, Stanford, CA, USA

Rosaura Perales, B.A. Palo Alto University, Palo Alto, CA, USA

David E. Reed II Palo Alto University, Palo Alto, CA, USA

Ruth V. Reed, MBBChir MRCPCH, MRCPsych Oxford Health NHS Foundation Trust, Warneford Hospital, Oxford, UK

John P. Rettger, Ph.D. Stanford Early Life Stress & Pediatric Anxiety Program, Stanford, CA, USA

Marilee Ruebsamen, Ph.D. Abbey Psychological Services, San Jose, CA, USA

Anna Staudenmeyer, M.S. Pacific Graduate School of Psychology, Palo Alto University, Palo Alto, CA, USA

Andrea Spear, M.A. Palo Alto University, Palo Alto, CA, USA

Paul J. Sullivan, M.S. Center for the Study and Treatment of Anxious Youth at Palo Alto University, Palo Alto University, Palo Alto, CA, USA

Micaela A. Thordarson, M.S. Center for the Study and Treatment of Anxious Youth at Palo Alto University, Palo Alto University, Palo Alto, CA, USA

Sandra Trafalis, Ph.D. Center for the Study and Treatment of Anxious Youth at Palo Alto University, Palo Alto University, Palo Alto, CA, USA

Rebecca Tyrer, B.Sc., M.Res. Leeds Teaching Hospitals NHS Trust, Leeds Institute of Health Sciences, Leeds, UK

Part I

Stressors for Immigrant Youth

Immigrant Youth Life Stressors

Anna Staudenmeyer, Erynn Macciomei,
Margareth Del Cid, and Sita G. Patel

Abstract

Although the relationship between stressors and psychopathology has been firmly established in adolescence, the heterogeneous context and characteristics of immigration, settlement, and reception confer specific stressors for immigrant youth above and beyond developmentally normal stressors faced by most youth. A conceptual model for understanding the relationship between stressful experiences and psychopathology in immigrant youth is crucial in order to implement effective treatment within this vulnerable population. This chapter defines immigrant youth life stressors as frequent environmental events or conditions that pose a risk to physical and psychological health and may compound the risk associated with previous trauma exposure. Based on a review of the literature, a categorization of immigrant youth life stressors is proposed. This chapter reviews and organizes research on immigrant youth and, based on the findings, advocates for a broader and more collaborative approach to treatment. A case example highlights how categorizing stressors holds clinical utility in guiding clinical case formulation and prioritizing intervention.

Keywords

Immigrant • Refugee • Youth • Stressors • Moderators • Mediators

Introduction

Research overwhelmingly affirms the relationship between stressful experiences and psychopathology across development. However, unanswered questions remain regarding how and when stressors predict mental health problems and trajectories

A. Staudenmeyer (✉) • E. Macciomei • M. Del Cid • S.G.Patel
Pacific Graduate School of Psychology, Palo Alto University, Palo Alto, CA, USA
e-mail: astudenmeyer@paloaltou.edu

© Springer International Publishing Switzerland 2016
S.G. Patel, D. Reicherter (eds.), *Psychotherapy for Immigrant Youth*,
DOI 10.1007/978-3-319-24693-2_1

toward developmental psychopathology on the one hand or resilience on the other [1]. Grant's widely accepted conceptual model for understanding the role of stressors in adolescent psychopathology proposes five basic tenets: (1) stressors predict psychopathology; (2) moderators alter the relationship between stressors and psychopathology; (3) stressors activate mediators which explain the relationship between stressors and psychopathology; (4) specificity exists in the associations between stressors, moderators, mediators, and psychopathology; and (5) reciprocal and dynamic relations occur among stressors, moderators, mediators, and psychopathology [2]. The informed development and advancement of primary, secondary, and tertiary mental health interventions require focused attention on the distinct variables that alter or explain the relationship between specific stressors and psychopathology in adolescents [2].

Nowhere is the need to apply a conceptual model for stressors as great as in the area of immigrant youth life stress. Data from the US Census Bureau's 2012 American Community Survey revealed that 25 % of all children under the age of 18 live with at least one immigrant parent. Of these children, 88 % are second-generation immigrants (born in the USA), and 12 % were first-generation immigrants (born outside of the USA). The heterogeneous context and characteristics of immigration, settlement, and reception confer specific stressors for immigrant youth above and beyond developmentally normal stressors faced by most youth [3]. Preexisting risk and protective factors for immigrant youth, such as premigration exposure to trauma, social support, and family intactness, may enhance or diminish the relationship between stressors and measures of adaptation. Furthermore, stressors arising from the experience of immigration can strain physical and emotional resources and challenge traditional problem-solving and coping strategies, which may in turn explain the relationship between stressors and outcomes. It is crucial to unpack the moderators and mediators of the stressors—psychosocial adaptation relationship in order to implement effective interventions within the vulnerable population of immigrant youth.

Extending beyond symptom-based outcomes to account for functioning in school, family, and peer contexts allows research on immigrant youth to be unbound by its traditional focus on psychopathology [4] and calls attention to the multiple domains in which immigrant youth face challenges that can be effectively targeted by intervention. A conceptual model of stressors for immigrant youth should reflect this need and investigate the role of stressors in the development of various psychosocial outcomes, representing a slight departure from the model posed by Grant and colleagues [2]. Addressing depression, anxiety, and posttraumatic stress disorder (PTSD) symptoms among immigrant youth would be incomplete and misinformed without a thorough inventory of sociocultural stressors faced by the youth, such as poverty, neighborhood violence, discrimination, intergenerational conflict, family separation, legal status, and language acquisition. Psychological interventions for immigrant youth must involve collaboration between the various systems and contexts to which the youth belongs (Table 1).

Table 1 Stressors and responses

Stressor	Excerpt
Poverty	I think not having to have a job is kind of stressful. Because, you know, my mom, she has to take care of a lot of people, like the whole family and plus my nephews and things like that, and she has to work and what she gets paid is not enough and she has to work extra. So it's kind of stressful cause I can't get a job cause you know, I'm illegal in here so it's hard for me to get a job.
Family separation	For me, something that is difficult is being here in this country and my grandma raised me. I wasn't raised by my mom. Right now she is back in Panama, where I was born and she's kind of sick right now and I want to go and see her. I can't so I feel kind of sad. But I have to deal with it.
Discrimination	We don't have the same cultures… they used to laugh at me…Even the teachers laugh at me like they show me some pictures in the books of old Africa and ask me if this is where I lived looks like this. You know…I didn't speak English, so…I only get mad inside.
Legal status	I am still waiting for my green card and I don't know how long it's going to take because I've been here 6 years and I haven't gotten my green card. I wrote them a letter and the process time is out and that worries me. I want my green card so I could go back to my native country and visit. I heard that some people go back to their country and they are not able to enter the USA again. I don't know. It's those legal things.
Language acquisition	It was really hard. I used to cry every single night when I went to like from the school they give us homework so I couldn't do it cause it was another language and I couldn't understand.

Definition and Categorization of Life Stressors

This chapter defines immigrant youth life stressors as environmental events or conditions [2], which are frequent [5]; pose a risk to physical, cognitive, and psychological health [6]; and may compound the risk posed by prior exposure to traumatic events [7]. Research detailing ongoing stress for immigrant youth adopts variable terminology, such as daily hassles, chronic stressors, and stressful live events. This overlap and inconsistency in utilized constructs has been reflected more broadly in stress literature [8]. Because different studies may use different terminology to refer to the same stressful experiences, the proposed definition of life stressors has been formulated to allow for a comprehensive examination of stressful experiences that immigrant youth face. This definition intentionally distinguishes between stressful and traumatic events, which is another aspect of immigrant youth experience warranting specific attention. As such, this book devotes a separate chapter to trauma within immigrant youth populations.

Immigrant youth life stressors have been categorized in the literature in three main ways: according to the particular domain in which the stressor takes place

[9, 10], according to the social conditions or acculturative realities facing immigrant youth [3, 11–17], and based on the chronological groupings of stressors within the immigration process [18]. This proposed categorization of stressors is not mutually exclusive; for example, a neighborhood stressor (domain) such as living in a high-crime area may also be a reflection of limited capital (sociocultural stressor), such as poverty, that is occurring post-migration (a chronological stressor). However, this categorization is offered as a clinical tool for conceptualizing and organizing stressors faced by immigrant youth. Below is an elaboration on each category of stressor with a focus on how this categorization may hold clinical utility.

Domain-Specific Stressors Immigrant youth life stressors can be understood as relating to particular domains, such as parents, peers, school, the self, leisure, romantic partner, the future, the neighborhood, and resources [9, 10]. The domain categorization of immigrant youth life stressors may hold relevance for clinicians, as it provides a snapshot of the specific areas that may be challenging to this population, and allows for comparisons by nativity and cultural background. Literature supporting the immigrant paradox or diminishing levels of well-being as a function of time in the USA often do not consider how particular domains of stressors may be different depending on generational status. Investigating this question cross-sectionally allows for comparisons between generations to be made at a single time point. One study found no differences in the number of reported school stressors between first-generation immigrants and native youth, yet found a comparatively higher number of school stressors reported by second-generation immigrants. First-generation immigrants reported more stressors related to parents, the self, leisure, romantic partners, and the future, whereas second-generation reported more stressors with respect to parents, school, and romantic partner [10].

Understanding how domains of stressors change for immigrant youth over time spent in the USA is of immediate relevance to education, health, and mental health professionals working or coming into contact with immigrant youth. One longitudinal study looked at changes in stressors across a 3-year period for Arab Muslim immigrant youth [9], a particularly understudied immigrant population [4, 17, 19]. The authors argued that Islamic cultural beliefs and values on the issues of parental role and gendered expectations of children might present unique patterns of stressors as compared to other immigrant youth groups [9]. Participants consisted of immigrant and refugee youth, ranging in ages from 11 to 15, and their mothers, some of whom were refugees. School stressors were the most frequently reported stressor across all three waves of data collection, followed by parent stressors. Overall, both parent stressors and school stressors increased over time, whereas peer and resource stressors (operationalized as material resources important to youth, such as nice clothes) declined over time. Neighborhood stressors reflecting crime and safety remained stable with time [9]. Contrary to the authors' hypotheses, there were no gender effects on stressors. Also unexpected was the finding that immigrant youth with refugee mothers reported fewer parent and peer stressors but more neighborhood stressors than youth without refugee mothers. The authors posited that youth with refugee mothers may feel the need to protect their parents by reporting less hassles. Peer-related stressors are common among adolescents and immigrant youth. Lower reported peer-related stressors might be a function of the ethnic density of Arab Muslim immigrants within the study area [9]. This study highlights the importance of studying trajectories of domain-related stressors within and across ethnic groups of immigrant youth.

Sociocultural Stressors The broad category of sociocultural stressors is used to subsume a wide array of immigrant youth stressors described in the literature. It should be noted that this designation operates as a heuristic and is not intended to conflate disparate stressors. Multiple bidirectional sociocultural realities shape the particular life stressors faced by immigrant youth. Poverty, neighborhood violence, parental education and employment, family separation, discrimination, school segregation, legal concerns, acculturation, language difficulties, and intergenerational conflict incur stress not generally faced by nonimmigrant youth. A series of studies by Patel and colleagues used qualitative interviews with newcomer immigrant youth to illustrate their first-hand experiences with sociocultural stressors [81, 82]. Although each excerpt has been selected to elucidate a specific stressor, the complexity and interactions between sociocultural factors become fully apparent.

Chronological Stressors Although research uses the first two categories of stressors for diverse samples of immigrant youth, the chronological categorization is often reserved for understanding stressors faced by refugees, a particularly vulnerable population within immigrant youth. The chronological framework can account for unique stressors associated with different time points in the immigration process [18]. Research on psychopathology and psychosocial adaptation in refugee populations has historically focused on premigration political violence and war trauma as predictors of mental health outcomes. In their synthesis of literature, Miller and Rasco [18] propose political violence and displacement-related stressors as two sets of stressors threatening mental health outcomes among refugees. The latter category includes: (1) pre-displacement experiences of trauma and loss that do not include political violence; (2) displacement stressors arising from the process of displacement itself, such as trauma or stress within refugee camps or during the process of migration; and (3) post-displacement factors reflecting stressful social conditions which refugees face, such as poverty, discrimination, fear of deportation, and acculturation difficulties [18, 20].

Displacement-related stressors comprise events and conditions occurring across a range of settings, time, and intensity. Research focusing only on the refugee experience of political violence neglects to account for important stressors at various stages in the process of displacement. Research findings may then over-attribute variance in psychological outcomes to premigration war trauma and overlook the role of stressors during and after displacement [18]. This trauma-focused perspective not only guided research but also carried, and continues to carry, implications for clinical interventions used to treat psychological symptomatology in refugee populations [20]. Increased investigation of the relationship between displacement-related stressors and psychosocial outcomes calls attention to the importance of assessing and managing post-displacement stressors as a part of mental health interventions for refugees.

Limitations of Research on Immigrant Youth Life Stressors and Psychopathology

Longitudinal studies have provided conclusive evidence that stressors predict internalizing and externalizing psychopathology in children and adolescents [1]. The prospective designs of these studies eliminated the potentially confounding effects of symptoms and stressors being measured simultaneously and allowed for changes in the relationship between stressors and mental health symptoms to be assessed over time, after controlling for prior levels of internalizing and externalizing symptoms [21]. Although prospective methodology may be considered the gold standard in establishing a confound-free understanding of the role of stressors on developmental psychopathology, this design has been less frequently employed in studies on immigrant youth populations.

The immigrant paradox broadly refers to the notion of worsening health outcomes with increasing length of residence in the host country. This theory largely stems from research on physical health outcomes (versus mental health outcomes) in treatment-seeking or clinical samples of immigrants. However, most research of generational differences and psychopathology has been conducted on adults. In general, research has indicated mixed results in relation to generational considerations. Some research highlights a greater incidence of psychopathology, particularly anxiety and depressive disorders, in first-generation immigrants when compared to their native-born peers [22]. Conversely, the immigrant paradox theorizes that longer time in the host country is associated with more negative outcomes, including mental health, academic, and risk behaviors [23]. This can easily become confounded with increasing rates of psychopathology and decreasing academic engagement that has been documented among all early adolescent youth, not just immigrants. More longitudinal studies are necessary to determine the relevance of this paradox for psychological symptoms and psychosocial outcomes in nonclinical samples of immigrant youth. Furthermore, mental health symptoms of immigrant youth are typically investigated within clinical samples, leaving many questions unanswered about symptomatology in immigrant youth who are not receiving treatment [14].

Application of Conceptual Model of Stressors to Immigrant Youth

Sociocultural Life Stressors Predict Psychosocial Outcomes Stressors have been found to predict negative psychosocial outcomes in adolescence, but this relationship has been studied less often in immigrant youth. Immigrant youth face additional stressors than their nonimmigrant counterparts. Socioeconomic status may constitute a set of contextual stressors existing for immigrant youth in addition to normative adolescent stressors. For example, in 2014 approximately 28 % of first-generation immigrant youth and 25 % of second-generation immigrant youth lived below the federal poverty threshold, compared to 19 % of nonimmigrant youth [24].

Acculturation represents a normative process of immigrants navigating and negotiating between familiar, native cultural values and new norms within a host country. Acculturative stress is a term characterizing the challenges and conflicts that may result when immigrants are faced with cultural differences between their native and host culture [25]. Aspects of acculturative stress for immigrant youth include learning new cultural norms and expectations, balancing the adoption of new host values with the relinquishment of native cultural values, and dealing with covert and/or overt instances of discrimination by the host culture [26].

Over the past decade, more focus has been given to the parallel and distinct process of enculturation, or the extent to which immigrants retain the dominant values, practices, and language of their culture of origin [27]. Gaps in levels of acculturation and enculturation between immigrant youth and their parents have been investigated as predictors of poor mental health outcomes and engagement in risk behaviors. High levels of acculturation and enculturation, also discussed in terms of biculturalism, have been studied as a protective factor against negative psychosocial adaptation in immigrant youth [15, 27].

In keeping with the general conceptual model put forth by Grant and colleagues [2], findings presented will be culled from prospective studies to reveal the role of various sociocultural stressors in trajectories of development. As more recent studies include various measures of psychosocial well-being as outcomes, such as psychological symptoms and academic difficulties, the same study may be presented in multiple outcomes sections below. Important risk and protective factors as well as mediators of sociocultural stressors will be highlighted.

Psychological Outcomes More focus has typically been given to understanding the relationship between stressors and psychopathology than other psychosocial outcomes. However, much of what is known about developmental outcomes in immigrant youth is gleaned from cross-sectional data, making it difficult to understand how the relationship between stressors and psychopathology changes with time [14], warranting a focus on prospective findings [2].

Internalizing Symptoms Internalizing symptoms have been examined as outcomes less often in immigrant youth literature than externalizing symptoms, which is in contrast to studies of psychopathology in nonimmigrant adolescents [1, 14]. The New York City Academic and Social Engagement Study (NYCASES) represents prospective efforts to investigate psychosocial trajectories of immigrant youth [28]. Results of NYCASES revealed that unlike trends in nonimmigrant youth samples, internalizing symptoms declined over the high school years. However, sociocultural stressors moderated this trend, with increasing levels of stressors leading to increases in anxiety, depression, and somatic symptoms [14]. Results of this study provide empirical evidence for the long-term effects of sociocultural stressors on mental health symptoms of immigrant youth.

Prospective results from the Latino Acculturation and Health Project provide a rich understanding of how and under what circumstances sociocultural stressors predict the development of mental health problems [15]. This longitudinal investigation involved nearly 350 immigrant youth and their parents. Over half of the sample of youth was first-generation immigrants, with the remainder being second-generation immigrants. Results from the Latino Acculturation and Health Project revealed a decrease in internalizing symptoms and an increase in self-esteem over the 2-year study period. After taking into account time spent in the USA, it was shown that increased length of residence was related to lower self-esteem scores in immigrant youth [15]. Sociocultural stressors emerged as more robust predictors of mental health outcomes (both internalizing symptoms and self-esteem) than measures of cultural identification.

A longitudinal study of 749 first- and second-generation Mexican immigrant youth and their families investigated how sociocultural stressors related to internalizing symptoms across time. The experience of language and discrimination stressors in 5th grade was related to greater internalizing symptoms in 7th grade [29]. Fluctuations in sociocultural stressors within a sample of first- and second-generation Mexican immigrant adolescent mothers predicted increases in their depressive symptoms one year later, even after controlling for baseline depressive symptoms and economic hardship [30]. These findings were relevant for within-person fluctuations as well as between-person fluctuations, making sociocultural stressors robust predictors of depressive symptoms in Mexican-origin mothers [30]

Another prospective study of first- and second-generation immigrant youth in Greece investigated the extent to which socioeconomic stressors in immigrant youth posed a risk for adaptation and psychological well-being [12]. Immigrant youth life stressors of immigrant status and socioeconomic stressors did not predict internalizing symptoms. This divergent finding poses interesting questions about the universality of immigrant youth life stress.

Externalizing Symptoms Immigrant status and socioeconomic stressors predicted conduct problems for youth in Greek public schools at baseline and were related to increases in conduct problems over time. This increase in externalizing symptoms was found among both immigrant and nonimmigrant youth [12]. Mexican immigrant youth who reported more language hassles in 5th grade experienced increases in externalizing symptoms between 5th and 7th grade [29].

Risk Behaviors Studies of risk behaviors in immigrant youth frequently assess the relationship of immigrant nativity with engagement in risky behaviors, such as substance use and sexual risk taking, largely providing evidence to support the immigrant paradox. A prospective investigation of a nationally representative sample of Latino immigrant youth found that first-generation youth were less likely than their second-generation peers to drink alcohol or smoke cigarettes or marijuana [31]. This relationship was mediated by perceived peer substance use in that US-born immigrant youth were more likely to associate with substance-using peers and reported higher levels of substance use after 1 year than foreign-born Latino youth. Both perceived peer substance use and school connectedness were directly associated with substance use, suggesting that school offers protective benefits to youth that are independent of peer affiliation [31]. Cross-sectional studies have also found that US-born Latino and Asian youth report engaging in more sex and drug risk behaviors than their foreign-born peers [32]. Although first-generation youth were more likely to abstain from alcohol and sex than second- and third-generation youth, the relative advantage of nativity disappeared by the third generation, where patterns of risk behaviors resembled non-Latino white youth [32]. Although there have been documented protective benefits against risk taking in foreign-born and recently arrived immigrant youth, it has been shown that this group has unique risk factors for future risk-taking behaviors. For example, immigrant youth residing in the USA for less than 6 years reported experiencing more social pressure to engage in risk behaviors while simultaneously receiving less parental support to abstain from these risk behaviors [33].

Less literature exists which prospectively examines how immigrant youth life stressors relate to engagement in risk behaviors [30]. Cross-sectional studies have documented an association between violence-related inner-city stressors and substance use behaviors in immigrant youth that remains significant after accounting for protective factors such as family cohesion [27]. A study of first- and second-generation Mexican adolescent mothers offered a longitudinal examination of how fluctuations in sociocultural stressors over time led to engagement in risk-taking behaviors, such as fighting, property damage, and alcohol and drug use. Results indicated that for mothers experiencing high levels of sociocultural stressors (specifically enculturative stressors) relative to the overall sample, fluctuations in enculturative stressors predicted increased engagement in risk activities [30]. This was not true for mothers reporting lower levels of enculturative stress relative to the overall sample.

Academic Outcomes When stressors among immigrant youth have been studied, outcomes have typically been bound to measures of psychopathology, with other developmentally relevant outcomes such as school performance receiving less focus [4, 17, 19]. Academic outcomes and engagement in risk behaviors are valuable indices of adjustment for immigrant youth. Research with low-income minority (nonimmigrant) adolescents examined the relationship between life stressors and grade point average (GPA) and found that more life stressors predicted lower GPA [3, 11]. Life stressors may also have a negative impact on academic achievement over time. For example, family stressors and academic stressors (operationalized as daily attendance, difficulties in understanding, and poor evaluations) in the 9th grade have been found to predict a decline in GPA over the course of high school for adolescents from Mexican, Chinese, and European backgrounds [34].

Motto-Stefanidi and colleagues [12] found that academic trajectories of GPA declined over time with both immigrant and nonimmigrant youth in Greek public schools. Other longitudinal studies have documented declining academic performance in immigrant youth [35]. The observed decline in both groups makes it difficult to attribute the worsening outcomes to immigration or acculturative stressors and further supports existing literature showing declines in academic performance across early adolescence, irrespective of immigrant status. Despite the overall negative trend in academic performance, more pronounced declines have been observed when the immigrant youth face more adversity and discrimination, which was not specifically measured in the study [12].

Moderators of Psychosocial Outcomes The lack of systematic investigation of moderators across studies precludes the ability to understand and target the connections that exist between stressors and psychosocial adaptation [36]. Consequently, this deficit has been a limitation of adolescent stress literature generally and immigrant youth stress literature specifically. Identifying moderators of the relationship between immigrant youth life stressors and psychosocial outcomes can help to design and implement effective psychosocial interventions for this population. At an individual level, moderators may also provide important information to clinicians, social workers, and teachers about an adolescent's level of risk for negative psychosocial outcomes. Below we present moderators of psychosocial outcomes that have been identified in limited longitudinal studies of immigrant youth life stressors.

Family cohesion, operationalized as family supportiveness, was found to moderate the relationship between language stressors and changes in symptom internalization over time for first-generation, but not second-generation, Mexican immigrant youth. No relationship existed between language stressors and internalizing symptoms when family cohesion was high for first-generation immigrant youth. When family cohesion was low, there was a significant relationship between language stressors and internalizing symptoms [29]. Family cohesion did not moderate the relationship between discrimination and mental health symptoms. Different studies have identified and explored other aspects of the family climate as moderators of mental health outcomes: When parental involvement and youth self-efficacy were taken into account, immigrant status and socioeconomic stressors of youth in Greek public schools were not significantly related to internalizing or externalizing symptoms [12]. Although parental involvement and youth self-efficacy offered some protection against symptoms of psychopathology, they did not buffer the effects of immigrant status and socioeconomic stressors on GPA [12]. The inability of social resources to afford protective academic benefits to stressed immigrant youth has also been documented in cross-sectional studies [3].

Research with immigrant youth often views social support as a moderator of mental health outcomes. Important moderators of the relationship between acculturative stressors and internalizing symptoms emerged from NYCASES. Social support networks conferred protection against the negative effects of acculturative stressors, such that more positive social support was associated with less withdrawn/depressed and anxious/depressed symptoms. Social support moderated the relationship between stressors and anxious/depressed symptoms in immigrant youth, serving as a buffer against the influence of acculturative stressors [28].

Neighborhood cohesion is a construct reflecting shared values, trust, and support for specific immigrant cultures among neighborhoods. Broadly speaking, neighborhood cohesion has been found to moderate the relationship between sociocultural stressors and mental health outcomes. The specific way that neighborhood cohesion served as a moderator differs by gender [29]. When neighborhood cohesion was low, language stressors were positively related to increasing trajectories of externalizing symptoms for boys. High neighborhood cohesion reversed the relationship between language stressors and externalizing symptoms for girls: Externalizing symptoms decreased despite language stressors for girls living in highly cohesive neighborhoods [29].

The American Psychological Association [37] has emphasized understanding the role of gender in psychosocial outcomes of immigrant youth, and a growing amount of research has incorporated analyses of gender differences. Inconsistent findings of gender as a moderator of mental health outcomes have been reported, with some of the evidence being drawn from cross-sectional studies. There is evidence to indicate gender differences in the report of internalizing symptoms among immigrant youth: Girls are more likely to report symptoms of anxiety [14] and depression [10, 14]. Another study also found that girls endorsed higher rates of internalizing symptoms and depression, whereas boys indicated higher rates of conduct problems [38]. However, there is also evidence showing that boys endorsed symptoms of depression and anxiety at higher rates than girls [13].

Level of enculturation and acculturation, operationalized and measured differently depending on the study, has been investigated as a moderator of the link between immigrant youth life stressors and psychosocial outcomes. For example, NYCASES looked at ethnic identification and US identification as moderators of mental health symptoms for Asian and Latino immigrant youth. Ethnic identity was found to afford protection against the development of mental health symptoms in immigrant youth exposed to acculturative stressors. Higher levels of ethnic identification in Asian and Latino youth were associated with lower withdrawn/depressed symptomatology [28]. Another prospective study of Latino immigrant youth found that ethnic identification predicted higher self-esteem, which may assist immigrant youth in coping with life stressors [15].

Youth's identification and involvement with US culture, or level of acculturation, has been an inconsistent predictor of mental health outcomes in immigrant youth. Within NYCASES, US identification did not predict internalizing symptoms in Asian and Latino immigrant youth [28]. However, in a sample of primarily foreign-born Latino immigrant youth, US cultural involvement predicted lower levels of internalizing symptoms [15]. The latter finding is consistent with literature relating low assimilation with poorer psychosocial outcomes.

Generational status (first versus second generation) emerged as a moderator of the relationship between immigrant status and psychosocial outcomes. Second-generation youth had increasing popularity and declining trajectories of externalizing behaviors over time compared to first-generation immigrant youth [12]. In another study, first-generation youth endorsed greater anxious and depressed symptomatology and more acculturative stress than second-generation youth [28]. In relation to psychological outcomes, second-generation Latino immigrants reported more mental health diagnoses than those of their first-generation counterparts [39]. Generational status has been studied as a moderator of academic performance and achievement. Generational status has been shown to impact academic performance of immigrant youth differentially, with second-generation immigrant youth having a more significant decline in GPA than first-generation youth [12]. Another study highlighted more negative academic outcomes and depression in later generations of immigrant adolescents [40]. These findings are generally in line with the concept of immigrant paradox.

Mediators Mediators of the relationship between stressors and psychosocial outcomes have been identified less in the literature. In a sample of primarily first-generation Latino immigrant youth, parent-adolescent conflict mediated the effects of acculturative stressors on psychological outcomes. More specifically, parent-adolescent conflict mediated the effects of acculturation conflicts and perceived discrimination on internalizing symptoms and self-esteem [15].

Some specific sociocultural stressors, such as perceived discrimination and acculturation conflicts, were more strongly related to mental health outcomes in cross-sectional analyses than longitudinal analyses. One hypothesis for this finding involves acculturative stressors being mediated by factors with stronger longitudinal effects, such as substance abuse, highlighting the need for more longitudinal research to uncover important mediators of the relationship between stressors and psychopathology [15].

Application of Conceptual Model of Stressors to Refugee Youth

Nearly 20 million children and adolescents worldwide have been forcibly displaced by conflict, with approximately a third of these individuals crossing international borders to seek refuge and asylum in new countries [41]. Exposure to war violence consistently predicts mental health problems among refugees under the age of 18 [41]. The trauma of these events can alter biological and psychological developmental trajectories long after exposure [42, 43]. Migration and relocation trauma often result in adverse psychological outcomes, particularly PTSD and depression [44–47]. Child refugees in the USA have an increased incidence of traumatic loss, exposure to violence, as well as academic, behavioral, and psychological problems [44]. Although prevalence rates of PTSD in refugee youth vary considerably, from 11 to 54 %, these are still higher than those of the general population, which ranges from 2 to 9 % [45, 48–53]. Premigration stressors predicted internalizing and externalizing symptoms and PTSD [48]. Those children who experienced direct physical injury or separation from parents also had higher rates of PTSD [51]. Rates of depression in refugee youth also varied considerably, from 3 to 30 % [45, 49, 52].

Research on psychopathology and psychosocial adaptation in refugee youth populations has historically adopted a trauma focus, exploring the relationship between pre-displacement trauma and mental health outcomes. This narrow research focus overlooks important stressors at various stages in the process of displacement. Research findings may then over-attribute variance in psychological outcomes to pre-displacement trauma and negate the role of stressors during and after resettlement [18]. Given the pronounced stressors facing immigrant and refugee youth, failing to consider how stressors relate to psychosocial outcomes or how they may change the relationship between pre-displacement trauma and psychosocial outcomes precludes an understanding of adaptation for this population. A large number of refugee youth have been exposed to premigration war trauma [41], and many immigrant youth also face post-displacement life stressors like language acquisition, acculturation problems, perceived discrimination, and socioeconomic problems [53]. Therefore, it is crucial to examine the relationship between war exposure, post-displacement immigrant life stressors, and psychological outcomes.

Post-displacement life stressors alter the relationship between war exposure and mental health outcomes in refugee youth [40, 45, 54, 55]. Research shows that life stressors can operate as mediators that account for this relationship [10, 56, 57], or as moderators that alter the relationship [58]. For example, a study of youth in Sri Lanka found that, after controlling for war and tsunami-related stressors, exposure to life stressors predicted more internalizing and externalizing symptoms [56]. Furthermore, life stressors associated with poverty were stronger predictors of PTSD than direct war or tsunami exposure, showing that major traumatic events were not the primary source of distress among Sri Lankan youth. In another study, war-exposed youth from Sierra Leone who also experienced more current life stressors had increased internalizing symptoms [54]. A study of Somali adolescent refugees in the USA found that acculturative stressors such as criticism for "becoming too American," parents working long hours, and perceived discrimination were significant predictors of PTSD symptoms, even after controlling for premigration cumulative trauma [45]. An understanding of how trajectories of mental health outcomes are shaped by premigration trauma and post-displacement life stressors will allow for the development of appropriate interventions for refugee youth.

However, less is known about how multiple stressors may predict academic outcomes among immigrant refugees. Some research cites school as the most important system that immigrant youth encounter following resettlement [59]. One study found that regardless of the number and nature of premigration traumas they experienced, Somali refugee youth who endorsed lower levels of depression and higher self-efficacy also reported greater attachment, commitment, involvement, and belief in their school [59]. Research highlights that youth face academic difficulties early after immigration [35] and, for a majority, a downward trajectory of academic performance [19]. In an ethnically diverse clinical sample of refugee youth exposed to premigration war trauma, difficulties with schoolwork and grades were prevalent among over half of the adolescents [44].

Unaccompanied Minors Unaccompanied minors (UAMs) comprise a vulnerable segment of refugee youth. UAMs are youth, under the age of 18, who have been separated from their parents while undergoing the immigration process [60]. Of the nearly 20 million refugee children and adolescents worldwide, it is estimated that 2–5 % are separated from their families and fall into the category of UAM [61]. Some evidence suggests that UAMs experience more negative outcomes and life stressors when compared to other immigrant youth [48]. For example, UAMs deal with additional stressors including permanent versus temporary accommodation status and living arrangements [62]. Compared to accompanied immigrant/refugee youth, refugee UAMs experienced a greater number of stressful life events [48] and report more PTSD symptoms [48, 62]. Even though both UAMs and their accompanied counterparts were equally likely to experience post-displacement stressors and psychological problems [62], UAMs were more likely to develop internalizing and externalizing symptoms, with younger UAMs being most vulnerable [62, 63]. However, age has inconsistently been associated with mental health problems among UAMs in other studies [64]. Gender and ethnic background have been identified as important predictors of psychological outcomes among UAMs [64].

Case Study

The case study below highlights the unique challenges faced by immigrant youth. While each individual's experiences may vary, youth often encounter stressors before, during, and after migration. We know that it is necessary to consider this full range of stressors in order to appropriately account for variance in psychological outcomes within this population [44, 56, 65–67]. Identifying and understanding stressors across one's migration experience holds immediate relevance for intervention with immigrant youth.

Lucia is a 17-year-old Mexican female who immigrated to the USA 1 year ago. In Mexico, she lived with her grandmother, aunt, younger brother, and cousins in a rural farming area. Her mother immigrated to the USA when Lucia was 6 years old, shortly after the birth of Lucia's brother. Although Lucia spoke to her frequently by telephone, she did not see her mother for 10 years following her mother's emigration from Mexico. Last year, after a significant amount of gang violence broke out in Lucia's town, the family decided it would be safest for Lucia to live with her mother in the USA, with the hope that her brother may also eventually immigrate.

Lucia's family paid a "coyote," an individual that guides undocumented people cross the US border from Mexico [68], to transport her across the Mexican border. She traveled with two other teens from a nearby town. During their journey, Lucia and her fellow travelers were physically assaulted and verbally maltreated by the coyotes. They received inadequate amounts of food and water and were exposed to unsanitary conditions. Once they arrived in the USA, Lucia was arrested and held in an overcrowded detention center with little privacy. She did not know anyone in this facility, as those she was traveling were placed in a different detention center. Lucia was detained for 1 month before being released into the care of her mother. She moved in with her mother, stepfather, and two step siblings (ages 18 months old and 3 years old) in an apartment in a large, urban city. She currently shares a small bedroom with the other children, but sleeps on the couch most nights so as to not disturb her siblings when she comes home late from work.

Lucia is happy to be reunited with her mother. However, she quickly realized that adapting to her new life would be a challenge. Lucia recently began attending twelfth grade at a local inner-city high school and has been placed in classes for students identified as English language learners. Lucia hoped that with the chance to attend high school, she would learn English more quickly and develop a skill set to use for a future career. Despite being placed in specialized classes, she still feels behind her peers and often feels discouraged about her ability to complete the large amounts of homework she is assigned. Lucia works 6 days a week from 6 p.m. to 2 a.m. as a restaurant dishwasher to help her family save for her brother's emigration from Mexico. Her full-time work schedule has posed an additional challenge to the completion of her school assignments. While at home, she frequently disagrees with her mother and stepfather about her household responsibilities, including the care of her two step siblings. She is unable to concentrate and is failing almost every class. She has been reprimanded for being late to work on many occasions, making her fear that she may lose her job and not be able to pay her brother's passage to the USA. Lucia was recently notified that she will need to hire a lawyer to help her prepare her immigration documents, which has been adding to her stress.

A teacher at Lucia's school noticed that her grades have plummeted since last semester, she is frequently absent due to illness, and she is often falling asleep in class. When her teacher questioned her about a late homework assignment, Lucia exploded with anger, reporting that she has too many responsibilities. Her teacher referred Lucia to psychotherapy for the current troubles she is experiencing.

In her initial evaluation with the therapist, Lucia reported feeling exhausted. She described having trouble completing her daily duties with respect to school, her job, and her family. Lucia discussed the many responsibilities that she holds and her guilt for not being able to fulfill all of them. She also shared that she cannot get the horrific images of the coyote brutally beating one of her fellow travelers out of her mind. She explained that the realities of her everyday life are more challenging than she expected and that she is beginning to lose hope of the life she imagined with her mother and brother together in the USA.

In accordance with the aims of the chapter, we will highlight the varying stressors experienced by Lucia and make specific note of how these stressors can and should be handled in the context of psychotherapy. We will not be discussing any possible risk, including harm to self or others, potential for child abuse, etc. However, as with any case, addressing any possible risk should be included in the clinician's initial assessment [69].

Before beginning treatment with Lucia, a clinician must first evaluate his or her ability to competently provide services to an individual of this cultural and linguistic background. Clinicians who are unfamiliar with serving immigrant or diverse cultural populations may under- or over-pathologize risk factors and diagnoses [70, 71]. Consultation and translation services may be required when working with immigrant youth and families and must be competently integrated into treatment [72, 73]. In this particular case, the client is not a native English speaker and her level of English proficiency is unclear. Therefore, any documents will likely require translation into the client and family's language of choice. Verbal translation should not be left to the youth or family members, as this can place unnecessary stress on the family translator, especially when the clinician is discussing sensitive or uncomfortable topics [74–76]. The use of untrained translators can also prompt significant ethical concerns [77]. For example, a clinician should never use the youth or any family member to describe the limits of confidentiality, given the fundamental importance of clearly and professionally articulating this nuanced ethical obligation [78]. Additionally, the youth or family member may not know the specialized vocabulary related to particular subject matter or may take liberties with translation that trained translators would not [77, 79]. In light of these considerations, only trained translators should be utilized for all translation services [78, 79].

As a reminder, we define immigrant youth life stressors as environmental events or conditions [2] which are frequent [5]; pose a risk to physical, cognitive, and psychological health [6]; and may compound the risk posed by prior exposure to traumatic events [7]. As highlighted previously, there are three major categories in which Lucia's stressors can be organized: domain specific, sociocultural, and chronological. Lucia experiences domain-specific stressors related to challenges with her family (both in the USA and Mexico), school, work, legal status, lack of resources, and limited peer support. When considering sociocultural stressors, poverty creates overwhelming stress to Lucia and her family. Because of limited financial resources, she must work many hours and help with the childcare of her younger siblings. We see from the vignette that Lucia experiences further sociocultural stressors, including intergenerational conflict, family separation and reunification, language difficulties, acculturation, and legal concerns. Finally, Lucia's immigration process highlights chronological stressors related to the trauma and family challenges she has endured in all phases of the immigration process.

The clinician should first identify and categorize Lucia's specific stressors. This organization allows for more precisely linking each presenting problems with targeted interventions and furthermore makes monitoring and tracking changes in stressors across time possible. When prioritizing stressors, it is important to not only consider the referral source, but also choose stressors that seem to be most contributing to the client's overall distress. The clinician should expect to work in conjunction with multiple systems in order to find the most effective ways to address and alleviate immigrant youth life stressors. Identifying community resources for Spanish speakers or English language learners in general may ease Lucia's stressors in school, including her English language acquisition. Because more life stressors have been found to be associated with lower GPA [3, 11], easing these stressors might allow Lucia to allocate more time to her academics and language abilities and potentially raise her GPA. Intervention efforts for stressors affecting Lucia's academic performance should be addressed promptly, as most immigrant youth experiencing academic difficulties are not able to improve their GPA by the time they graduate [19].

Through the clinician collaborating with community agencies, Lucia may also be able to broaden her community network. Given that social support is a moderator of mental health outcomes [26], this may aid in mitigating some of her symptoms. Building social support may also be particularly culturally relevant in the case of Lucia, being from a collectivist culture [80]. Through linking her family to resources such as low-income housing, free or low-cost child care, food bank services, free or low-cost legal services for immigrant children, and counseling services for immigrant families, financial strain on Lucia and her family may decrease, and family cohesion and parental involvement may increase. This assistance may allow Lucia to work fewer hours and may even afford the family the ability to more quickly save for the passage of Lucia's brother to the USA. Connecting immigrant youth and often their families to broader community resources allows the clinician to act as an advocate and collaborate with various systems and enables the clinician to focus his or her intervention efforts on the psychological concerns of the case.

When reading the vignette, Lucia's trauma history and depression, anxiety, and PTSD symptoms may have been particularly salient and concerning to readers who are trained clinicians. Before immediately moving to address the psychological concerns, Lucia's psychological symptoms should be reassessed. Because stressors predict psychopathology [2], it is possible that by aiding Lucia to alleviate these stressors, her symptoms of depression and anxiety may have decreased. This means that, through mitigating the stressors, her symptoms may begin to lessen without formal psychological intervention. The implementation of psychological interventions among immigrant youth would be incomplete and misinformed without first addressing stressors.

However, different prioritization may be required, depending on the stressors and presentation of the youth. This may be particularly relevant for clinicians working with youth who have been exposed to premigration war trauma and violence. For example, if the youth's functioning is dramatically impaired by his or her psychological symptoms, laying the groundwork for trauma-focused treatment sooner may be indicated. Additionally, there may be instances in which the order that stressors are addressed varies. For example, if there is a stressor that prompts particular urgency (such as a legal deadline) or is identified as particularly important to the individual, then those might be addressed first. While the model poses suggestions for clinicians to use when working with immigrant youth, clinicians should always use their best judgment.

Conclusion

Psychotherapy must be considered an interdependent, versus independent, intervention among immigrant youth. Compartmentalization of psychosocial services for immigrant youth, particularly refugees and UAMs, poses a barrier to the promotion of well-being and adaptation in this vulnerable and resilient population. Social service centers for UAMs often lack employees trained in being sensitive to the psychosocial needs of immigrant youth and may exacerbate the legal and residential stressors they face. Addressing depression, anxiety, and PTSD symptoms among immigrant youth would be incomplete and misinformed without a thorough inventory of sociocultural stressors faced by the youth, such as poverty, neighborhood violence, discrimination, intergenerational conflict, family separation, legal status, and language acquisition. Trauma-focused treatments for refugee youth with pre-displacement exposure to war and violence may need to be prioritized differently depending on the life stressors faced by the youth. These stressors may need to be logistically addressed (if possible) before beginning traditional trauma treatments.

The school emerges as a critical context for screening and intervention with immigrant youth. Guidance counselors, social workers, teachers, and school nurses possess valuable roles in mitigating the impact of school stressors and sociocultural stressors on mental health outcomes. Using one of the three proposed categories to chart changes in stressors when working individually with immigrant youth can be a tool for anticipating fluctuations in risk for adverse psychosocial outcomes, such as increased psychopathology, poor academic outcomes, and engagement in risk behaviors. Newcomer immigrant youth face unique stressors and may receive greater amounts of pressure to assimilate into mainstream culture than immigrant youth who have been in the country longer. This can be coupled with less parental awareness or encouragement to avoid risk behaviors. Interventions should be geared toward this early critical period of acculturation and include the parents of immigrant youth.

References

1. Grant KE, McMahon SD, Carter JS, Carleton RA, Adam EK, Chen E. The influence of stressors on the development of psychopathology. In: Lewis M, Rudolph KD, editors. Handbook of developmental psychopathology. 3rd ed. New York, NY: Springer; 2014. p. 205–24.
2. Grant KE, Compas BE, Stuhlmacher AF, Thurm AE, McMahon SD, Halpert JA. Stressors and child and adolescent psychopathology: moving from markers to mechanisms of risk. Psychol Bull. 2003;129(3):447–66. doi:10.1037/0033-2909.129.3.447.
3. Gillock KL, Reyes O. Stress, support, and academic performance of urban, low-income, Mexican-American adolescents. J Youth Adolesc. 1998;28(2):259–82.
4. Suárez-Orozco C, Carhill A, Chuang SS. Immigrant children: making a new life. In: Chuang SS, Moreno RP, editors. Immigrant children: change, adaptation, and cultural transformation. Lanham, MD: Lexington Books; 2010. p. 7–26.
5. Pratt LI, Barling J. Differentiating between daily events, acute and chronic stressors: a framework and its implications. In: Hurrell Jr JJ, Murphy LR, Sauter SL, Cooper CL, editors. Occupational stress: issues in research and development. Philadelphia, PA: Taylor and Francis; 1988. p. 41–53.
6. Sapolsky RM. Why zebras don't get ulcers: the acclaimed guide to stress, stress-related diseases, and coping. New York: Henry Holt and Company; 2004.
7. Kubiak SP. Trauma and cumulative adversity in women of a disadvantaged social location. Am J Orthopsychiatry. 2005;75(4):451–65.
8. Hahn SE, Smith CS. Daily hassles and chronic stressors: conceptual and measurement issues. Stress Med. 1999;15:89–101.
9. Aroian KJ, Templin TN, Hough ES. Longitudinal study of daily hassles in adolescents in Arab Muslim immigrant families. J Immigr Minor Health. 2014;16:831–8. doi:10.1007/s10903-013-9795-7.
10. Stefanek E, Strohmeier D, Fandrem H, Spiel C. Depressive symptoms in native and immigrant adolescents: the role of critical life events and daily hassles. Anxiety Stress Coping. 2012;25(2):201–17.
11. Dubois DL, Felner RD, Brand S, Adan AM, Evans EG. A prospective study of life stress, social support, and adaptation in early adolescence. Child Dev. 1992;63:542–57.
12. Motto-Stefanidi F, Asendorpf JB, Masten AS. The adaptation and well-being of adolescent immigrants in Greek schools: a multilevel, longitudinal study of risks and resources. Dev Psychopathol. 2012;24:451–73.
13. Oppedal B, Røysamb E. Mental health, life stress and social support among young Norwegian adolescents with immigrant and host national background. Scand J Psychol. 2004;45:131–44.
14. Sirin SR, Ryce P, Gupta T, Rogers-Sirin L. The role of acculturative stress on mental health symptoms for immigrant adolescents: a longitudinal investigation. Dev Psychol. 2013;49(4):736–48.
15. Smokowski PR, Rose RA, Bacallao ML. Influence of risk factors and cultural assets on Latino adolescents' trajectories of self-esteem and internalizing symptoms. Child Psychiatry Hum Dev. 2010;41(2):133–55.
16. Suárez-Morales L, Lopez B. The impact of acculturative stress and daily hassles on preadolescent psychological adjustment: examining anxiety symptoms. J Prim Prev. 2009;30: 335–49.
17. Suárez-Orozco C, Gaytan FX, Bang HJ, Pakes J, O'Connor E, Rhodes J. Academic trajectories of newcomer immigrant youth. Dev Psychol. 2010;46(3):602–18. doi:10.1037/a0018201.
18. Miller KE, Rasco LM. An ecological framework for addressing the mental health needs of refugee communities. In: Miller KE, Rasco LM, editors. The mental health of refugees: ecological approaches to healing and adaptation. London: Lawrence Erlbaum; 2004.

19. Suárez-Orozco C, Bang HJ, Onaga M. Contributions to variations in academic trajectories amongst recent immigrant youth. Int J Behav Dev. 2010;34(6):500–10. doi:10.1177/0165025409360304.
20. Miller KE, Rasmussen A. War exposure, daily stressors, and mental health in conflict and post-conflict settings: bridging the divide between trauma-focused and psychosocial frameworks. Soc Sci Med. 2010;70(1):7–16. doi:10.1016/j.socscimed.2009.09.029.
21. Grant KE, Compas BE, Thurm AE, McMahon SD, Gipson PY. Stressors and child and adolescent psychopathology: measurement issues and prospective effects. J Clin Child Adolesc Psychol. 2004;33(2):412–25.
22. Lustig SL, Kia-Keating M, Knight WG, Geltman P, Ellis H, Kinzie JD, Keane T, Saxe GN. Review of child and adolescent refugee mental health. J Am Acad Child Adolesc Psychiatry. 2004;43(1):24–36.
23. García-Coll C, Marks A, editors. The immigrant paradox in children and adolescents: Is becoming American a developmental risk? Washington, DC: American Psychological Association; 2011.
24. Child Trends. Immigrant children; 2014. Retrieved from http://www.childtrends.org/?indicators=immigrant-children-sthash.BQBQK7tl.dpuf
25. Berry JW. Immigration, acculturation, and adaptation. Appl Psychol. 1997;46(1):5–34.
26. Berry JW, Phinney JS, Sam DL, Vedder P. Immigrant youth: acculturation, identity, and adaptation. Appl Psychol. 2006;55(3):303–32.
27. Ramirez Garcia JI, Manongdo JA, Cruz-Santiago M. The family as mediator of the impact of parent-youth acculturation/enculturation and inner-city stressors on Mexican American youth substance use. Cult Divers Ethn Minor Psychol. 2010;16(3):404–12.
28. Rogers-Sirin L, Ryce P, Sirin SR. Acculturation, acculturative stress, and cultural mismatch and their influences on immigrant children and adolescents' well-being. In: Dimitrova R, Bender M, van de Vijver F, editors. Global perspectives on well-being in immigrant families. New York, NY: Springer; 2014. p. 11–30.
29. Nair RL, White RMB, Roosa MW, Zeiders KH. Cultural stressors and mental health symptoms among Mexican Americans: a prospective study examining the impact of the family and neighborhood context. J Youth Adolesc. 2012;42:1611–23.
30. Zeiders KH, Umana-Taylor AJ, Updegraff KA, Jahromi LB. An idiographic and nomothetic approach to the study of Mexican-origin adolescent mothers' socio-cultural stressors and adjustment. Prev Sci. 2015;16(3): 386–396.
31. Prado G, Huang S, Schwartz SJ, Maldonado-Molina MM, Bandiera FC, de la Rosa M, Pantin H. What accounts for differences in substance use among U.S.-born and immigrant Hispanic adolescents?: results from a longitudinal prospective cohort study. J Adolesc Health. 2009;45(2):118–25.
32. Hussey JM, Hallfors DD, Waller MW, Iritani BJ, Halpern CT, Bauer DJ. Sexual behavior and drug use among Asian and Latino adolescents: association with immigrant status. J Immigr Minor Health. 2007;9:85–94.
33. Blake SM, Ledsky R, Goodenow C, O'Donnell L. Recency of immigration, substance use, and sexual behavior among Massachusetts adolescents. Am J Public Health. 2001;91(5):794–8.
34. Flook L, Fuligni AJ. Family and school spillover in adolescents' daily lives. Child Dev. 2008;79(3):776–87.
35. Suárez-Orozco C, Rhodes J, Milburn M. Unraveling the immigrant paradox: academic engagement and disengagement among recently arrived immigrant youth. Youth Soc. 2009;41(2):151–85. doi:10.1177/0044118X09333647.
36. Grant KE, Behling S, Gipson PY, Ford RE. Adolescent stress: the relationship between stress and mental health problems. Prev Res. 2005;12(3):1–4.
37. American Psychological Association, Presidential Task Force on Immigration. Crossroads: the psychology of immigration in the new century; 2012. Retrieved from http://www.apa.org/topics/immigration/report.aspx
38. Nielsen SS, Norredam M, Christiansen KL, Obel C, Hilden J, Krasnik A. Organisational factors influencing asylum-seeking children's mental health. BMC Public Health. 2008;8:293.
39. Alegria M, Canino G, Shrout PE, Woo M, Duan N, Vila D, Torres M, Chen CN, Meng X. Prevalence of mental illness in immigrant and nonimmigrant U.S. Latino groups. Am J Psychiatry. 2008;165:359–69. doi:10.1176/appi.ajp.2007.07040704.

40. Kim YM, Newhill C, López F. Latino acculturation and perceived educational achievement: evidence for a bidimensional model of acculturation among Mexican-American children. J Hum Behav Soc Environ. 2013;23(1):37–52.
41. Fazel M, Reed RV, Panter-Brick C, Stein A. Mental health of displaced and refugee children resettled in high-income countries: Risk and protective factors. Lancet. 2012;379:266–82. doi:10.1016/S0140-6736(11)60051-2.
42. Mares S, Jureidini J. Psychiatric assessment of children and families in immigration detention — clinical, administrative and ethical issues. Aust N Z J Public Health. 2004;28(6):520–6.
43. Teicher MH, Andersen SL, Polcari A, Anderson CM, Navalta CP, Kim DM. The neurobiological consequences of early stress and childhood maltreatment. Neurosci Biobehav Rev. 2003;27(1):33–44.
44. Betancourt TS, Newnham EA, Layne CM, Kim S, Steinberg AM, Ellis H, Birman D. Trauma history and psychopathology in war-affected refugee children referred for trauma-related mental health services in the United States. J Trauma Stress. 2012;25:682–90. doi:10.1002/jts.21749.
45. Ellis BH, MacDonald HZ, Lincoln AK, Cabral HJ. Mental health of Somali adolescent refugees: the role of trauma, stress, and perceived discrimination. J Consult Clin Psychol. 2008;76(2):184–93. doi:10.1037/0022-006X.76.2.184.
46. Barowsky EI, McIntyre T. Migration and relocation trauma of young refugees and asylum seekers: Awareness as prelude to effective intervention. Child Educ. 2010;86(3):161–8. doi:10.1080/00094056.2010.10523138.
47. Bronstein I, Montgomery P. Psychological distress in refugee children: a systematic review. Clin Child Fam Psychol Rev. 2011;14:44–56. doi:10.007/s10567-010-0081-0.
48. Bean T, Derluyn I, Eurelings-Bontekoe E, Broekaert E, Spinhoven P. Comparing psychological distress, traumatic stress reactions, and experiences of unaccompanied refugee minors with experiences of adolescents accompanied by parents. J Nerv Ment Dis. 2007;195(4):288–97.
49. Heptinstall E, Sethna V, Taylor E. PTSD and depression in refugee children: associations with pre-migration trauma and post-migration stress. Eur Child Adolesc Psychiatry. 2004;13(6):373–80. doi:10.1007/s00787-004-0422-y.
50. Fazel M, Wheeler J, Danesh J. Prevalence of serious mental disorder in 7000 refugees resettled in western countries: a systematic review. The Lancet. 2005;365:1309–14.
51. Geltman PL, Grant-Knight W, Mehta SD, Lloyd-Travaglini C, Lustig S, Landgraf JM, Wise PH. The "lost boys of Sudan": functional and behavioral health of unaccompanied refugee minors resettled in the United States. Arch Pediatr Adolesc Med. 2005;159(6):585–91.
52. Hodes M, Jagdev D, Chandra N, Cunniff A. Risk and resilience for psychological distress amongst unaccompanied asylum seeking adolescents. J Child Psychol Psychiatry. 2008;49(7):723–32.
53. Porter M, Haslam N. Predisplacement and postdisplacement factors associated with mental health of refugees and internally displaced persons: a meta-analysis. J Am Med Assoc. 2005;294(5):602–12.
54. Gonzales NA, George PE, Fernandez AC, Huerta VL. Minority adolescent stress and coping. Prev Res. 2005;12(3).
55. Betancourt TS, McBain R, Newnham EA, Brennan RT. Trajectories of internalizing problems in war-affected Sierra Leonean youth: examining conflict and postconflict factors. Child Dev. 2013;84(2):455–70.
56. Ehntholt KA, Yule W. Practitioner review: assessment and treatment of refugee children and adolescents who have experienced war-related trauma. J Child Psychol Psychiatry. 2006;47(12):1197–210. doi:10.1111/j.1469-7610.2006.01638.x.
57. Fernando GA, Miller KE, Berger DE. Growing pains: the impact of disaster-related and daily stressors on the psychological and psychosocial functioning of youth in Sri Lanka. Child Dev. 2010;81(4):1192–210.
58. Rasmussen A, Nguyen L, Wilkinson J, Vundla S, Raghavan S, Miller KE, Keller AS. Rates and impact of trauma and current stressors among Darfuri refugees in eastern Chad. Am J Orthopsychiatry. 2010;80(2):227–36. doi:10.1111/j.1939-0025.2010.01026.x.

59. Miller KE, Omidian P, Rasmussen A, Yaqubi A, Daudzai H. Daily stressors, war experiences, and mental health in Afghanistan. Transcult Psychiatry. 2008;45(4):611–38. doi:10.1177/1363461508100785.
60. Kia-Keating M, Ellis BH. Belonging and connection to school in resettlement: young refugees, school belonging, and psychosocial adjustment. Clin Child Psychol Psychiatry. 2007;12:29–43.
61. UNHCR. UNHCR statistical yearbook. Geneva: UNHCR; 2001.
62. Derluyn I, Broekaert E. Unaccompanied refugee children and adolescents: the glaring contrast between a legal and a psychological perspective. Int J Law Psychiatry. 2008;31:319–30.
63. Michelson D, Sclare I. Psychological needs, service utilization, and provision of care in a specialist mental health clinic for young refugees: a comparative study. Clin Child Psychol Psychiatry. 2009;14(2):273–96.
64. Sourander A. Behavior problems and traumatic events of unaccompanied refugee minors. Child Abuse Negl. 1998;22(7):719–27.
65. Seglem KB, Oppedal B, Raedar S. Predictors of depressive symptoms among resettled unaccompanied refugee minors. Scand J Psychol. 2011;52:457–64.
66. Al-Krenawi A, Lev-Wiesel R, Mahmud AS. Psychological symptomatology among Palestinian adolescents living with political violence. Child Adolesc Mental Health. 2008;12(1):27–31. doi:10.1111/j.1475-3588.2006.00416.x.
67. Miller KE, Fernando GA, Berger DE. Daily stressors in the lives of Sri Lankan youth: a mixed methods approach to assessment in a context of war and natural disaster. Intervention. 2009;7(3):187–203.
68. Thabet AA, Vostanis P. Post traumatic stress disorder reactions in children of war: a longitudinal study. Child Abuse Negl. 2000;24(2):291–8.
69. O'Leary AO. Undocumented immigrants in the United States: an encyclopedia of their experience. Santa Barbara, CA: Greenwood; 2014.
70. Sommers-Flanagan J, Sommers-Flanagan R. Clinical interviewing. 4th ed. Hoboken, NJ: Wiley; 2009.
71. Matsumoto D, Juang L. Culture and psychology. 3rd ed. Belmont, CA: Wadsworth/Thomson Learning; 2004.
72. Pomerantz AM. Clinical psychology: science, practice, and culture: DSM-5 update. 3rd ed. Thousand Oaks, CA: Sage; 2014.
73. Bernal G, Sáez-Santiago E. Culturally centered psychosocial interventions. J Community Psychol. 2006;34(2):121–32. doi:10.1002/jcop.20096.
74. Sue S, Zane N, Nagayama Hall GC, Berger LK. The case for cultural competency in psychotherapeutic interventions. Annu Rev Psychol. 2009;60(1):525–48. doi:10.1146/annurev. psych60.110707.163651.
75. Katz V. Children as brokers of their immigrant families' health-care connections. Soc Probl. 2014;61(2):194–215. doi:10.1525/sp.2014.12026.
76. Morales A, Yakushko OF, Castro AJ. Language brokering among Mexican-immigrant families in the Midwest: a multiple case study. Couns Psychol. 2012;40(4):520–53. doi:10.1177/ 0011000011417312.
77. Rainey VR, Flores V, Morrison RG, David E, Silton RL. Mental health risk factors associated with childhood language brokering. J Multiling Multicult Dev. 2014;35(5):463–78. doi:10.10 80/01434632.2013.870180.
78. Bauer AM, Alegría M. Impact of patient language proficiency and interpreter service use on the quality of psychiatric care: a systematic review. Psychiatr Serv. 2010;61(8):765–73. doi:10.1176/appi.ps.61.8.765.
79. Searight HR, Searight BK. Working with foreign language interpreters: recommendations for psychological practice. Prof Psychol Res Pr. 2009;40(5):444–51. doi:10.1037/a0016788.
80. Morales A, Hanson WE. Language brokering: an integrative review of the literature. Hisp J Behav Sci. 2005;27(4):471–503. doi:10.1177/0739986305281333.
81. Patel SG, Tabb KM, Strambler MJ, Eltareb F. Newcomer immigrant adolescents and ambiguous discrimination the role of cognitive appraisal. J Adolesc Res. 2015;30(1):7–30.
82. Patel SG, Clarke AV, Eltareb F, Macciomei EE, Wickham R. Newcomer immigrant adolescents: a mixed-methods examination of family stressors and school outcomes. Sch Psychol Q. 2016;31(2):163–80.

Part II

**Psychotherapy Interventions
for Immigrant Youth**

Cognitive-Behavioral Therapy for Immigrant Youth: The Essentials

Micaela A. Thordarson, Marisa Keller, Paul J. Sullivan, Sandra Trafalis, and Robert D. Friedberg

Abstract

Cognitive-behavioral therapy (CBT) successfully treats a number of different emotional troubles youth experience. Though effectiveness studies with immigrant youth remain limited, the literature in existence reveals promising results for the treatment of immigrant youth with CBT. Modular CBT is a comprehensive treatment protocol specifically designed to flexibly address a variety of symptom clusters as well as attend to contextual psychosocial factors. In order to be potent, clinicians who practice must remain faithful to the cognitive-behavioral model and ground all interventions in the theoretical underpinnings. Case conceptualization represents the fundamental process that must be executed in order to understand the patient's particular presentation, identify crucial targets of treatment, and guide interventions along the way. This chapter thoroughly defines and illustrates content and process factors that comprise competent CBT for immigrant youth. Confabulated clinical examples are included throughout to depict in detail the ways that CBT is mildly modified to address cultural factors salient to practice with immigrant youth.

Keywords

Immigrant • Children • Adolescents • Youth • CBT • Modular CBT

All clinical examples contained in this chapter are de-identified and confabulated.

M.A. Thordarson • M. Keller • P.J. Sullivan • S. Trafalis
Center for the Study and Treatment of Anxious Youth, Palo Alto University,
Los Altos, CA 94022, USA

R.D. Friedberg (✉)
Center for the Study and Treatment of Anxious Youth, Palo Alto University,
Los Altos, CA 94022, USA

Center for the Study and Treatment of Anxious Youth, Palo Alto University,
5150 El Camino Real Ste. C-22, Los Altos, CA 94022, USA
e-mail: rfriedberg@paloaltou.edu

© Springer International Publishing Switzerland 2016
S.G. Patel, D. Reicherter (eds.), *Psychotherapy for Immigrant Youth*,
DOI 10.1007/978-3-319-24693-2_2

CBT with Immigrant Youth

Cognitive-behavioral therapy (CBT) is widely considered the most effective treatment for most childhood disorders. Until recently, however, the vast majority of empirical research was conducted with Caucasian youth of middle to upper socio-economic status. The last two decades witnessed a dramatic increase in the research focusing on whether established psychosocial treatments are successful with immigrant and/or ethnic minority youth [1–4]. CBT is identified as a psychosocial intervention that works effectively for ethnic minority and immigrant youth with minimal modification to standard treatment [1, 3, 5]. The radical transformations that accompany immigration often elicit significant distress from youth as they learn to integrate into a new home [6, 7]. Research on CBT among immigrant youth is sparse, but also suggests CBT successfully treats distress these patients face [2, 3, 8].

This chapter briefly introduces the theoretical framework of CBT and the literature supporting its effectiveness with immigrant youth. Essential ingredients to deliver competent CBT are then outlined. Modular CBT, a cutting-edge format of CBT that emphasizes flexibility and underscores the need for individualization of treatment, is described. Modular CBT is composed of several modules that are utilized in a progressive manner, driven by the case conceptualization of the patient's distress. Within each module are a variety of theoretically sound interventions that address different aspects of the patient's pathology (e.g., cognitive restructuring targets maladaptive thoughts). This format allows clinicians to conduct therapy in a manner specifically tailored to individual immigrant youth and the unique challenges they face (e.g., loss of social support, discrimination, economic struggles, fears of deportation, and learning new cultural norms [6]). Throughout the chapter, readers are provided with confabulated case examples to illustrate various clinical techniques and the manner in which interventions are designed to attend to immigrant needs.

Cognitive Behavior Therapy Model

Theoretical Foundations CBT integrates social learning theory, operant and classical conditioning, information processing, and cognitive theories [9, 10]. This comprehensive theoretical framework aims to alter maladaptive behavior patterns through changes in youths' thoughts, emotions, and physiological responses [10]. Goals are targeted through experiential learning, allowing young patients to learn by doing [10].

Empirical Support Available studies indicate immigrant youth will likely benefit from CBT in the same ways as nonimmigrant American youth [11–14]. Demographic characteristics such as age, gender, ethnicity, and symptom severity do not impact CBT's effectiveness [1, 5, 15, 16]. The past 20 years produced studies that support the use of CBT to treat youth who present to treatment for anxiety (e.g., [15, 17]), depression (e.g., [18]), posttraumatic stress disorder (e.g., [19]), disruptive behavior (e.g., [20, 21]), and challenges associated with autism spectrum disorder (e.g., [22–24]), substance use disorders (e.g., [25]), and eating disorders (e.g., [26]). CBT is an effective treatment model appropriate for youth for a wide range of presenting problems and cultural identities.

Appropriateness for Immigrant Youth CBT is an indicated intervention for immigrant youth. As discussed elsewhere in this book, studies introducing the use of CBT in schools with immigrant children reveal significant symptom reduction and enhanced functioning [2, 7, 27]. The empirical emphasis of CBT eliminates stigma often associated with therapy and encourages immigrant youth to identify the specific data that reflect distress—and growth [28, 29]. Emphasis on data collection allows cultural explanations of illness and idioms of distress to be expressed idiosyncratically, a facet providing much-needed flexibility when working with immigrant youth [11]. Collaboration and transparency imbue immigrant patients with much-needed empowerment [29].

Cognitive exercises can be used to identify attribution of discrimination and deconstruct perceived implications. Patel et al. [30] revealed such cognitive mechanisms influence severity of internalizing symptoms. A focus on concrete skills training gives immigrant youth and their families' specific strategies to help themselves, imbuing them with greater self efficacy [3, 28, 29]. Regardless of the country and culture of origin, research finds that CBT reduces symptoms of psychopathology and improves global functioning in immigrant youth and their families—whether they are experiencing anxiety, depression, posttraumatic stress, or other forms of psychopathology [2, 3, 27–29, 31]. Overwhelmingly, as researchers continue to investigate practice of CBT with ethnic minorities in general and immigrants in particular, results reflect the universal applicability and effectiveness of CBT for these youth.

Despite these very encouraging results, evaluating differences in treatment outcome provides only partial answers. For example, Cardemil [12] argues persuasively that no differences in outcome between culturally adapted and standard treatments are likely since the best culturally adapted programs maintain fidelity to the cognitive-behavioral models. Essentially, these comparative studies are evaluating very similar core elements. Consequently, examining differences in attrition rate and treatment involvement is more informative than symptom reduction alone. Indeed, Cardemil stated that cultural adaptations produce lower attrition rates and greater patient involvement in treatment among ethnic minority patients. Thus, if the particular cultural alteration (e.g., including extended family in sessions or predominantly targeting physiological symptoms rather than including cognitive) keeps more children in treatment and offers equivalent effectiveness, the change represents a good standard of care.

Based on the current literature, several recommendations emerge for working with immigrant youth. First, empirically supported treatments should be considered the first line of treatment for immigrant youth [1–3, 31, 32]. Simply, diverse groups of children profit from good CBT. Cultural adaptations should be considered and implemented, based on functional analysis, case formulation, and treatment planning [5, 10, 12, 31]. Treatment with any population must toe the line between faithfully implementing an evidence-based protocol and flexibly tailoring the intervention to the unique needs of an individual patient [33].

Modular CBT is one particularly flexible evidence-based treatment that lends itself to cultural adaptation [32]. Modularity allows the clinician to integrate various individual traits and experiences, including cultural variables [32]. However, it is important to remember that cultural adaptations that alter critical elements of the intervention fail to remain faithful to the empirically supported protocol [12]. In fact, when core components of an intervention are diluted or altered in the process of cultural adaptation, the resulting changes can have a deleterious effect on treatment outcome [34]. In other words, cultural adaptation must preserve the core treatment ingredients while allowing for flexible integration of diverse perspectives and values.

Essentials

CBT is an empirically valid therapy that delivers well-established, positive treatment outcomes for a number of diagnostic categories. The essential ingredients necessary for training clinicians to deliver CBT are the subject of much discussion in the literature [35, 36]. Friedberg and McClure [10] identified flexible application of protocols, case conceptualization, an active therapeutic stance, and session structure as integral skills for the child CBT clinician's toolbox. The following sections review each of these indispensable proficiencies. This section delineates the step-by-step content of CBT from the process factors that distinguish true CBT from mechanical execution of a manual.

Flexibility Within Fidelity

A common misunderstanding of CBT is that it is a rigid treatment protocol with little room for individualization to patients' needs. CBT protocols operationalize a treatment; however, they are not unyielding mandates [33]. CBT encourages flexible application to fit with the presenting problems of each patient. Kendall and colleagues [37] warn clinicians that there is a difference between flexibility and nonadherence to treatment. Adherence is vital as failure to remain faithful to CBT principles renders treatment ineffective. The literature implies that personalized treatments lead to better therapeutic outcomes [38].

The Coping Cat program is an exemplar of a manual-based program for anxious youth that embraces flexible application while remaining loyal to the core procedures of CBT [39]. In Coping Cat, Kendall and Hedtke execute the FEAR plan by individualizing progressive muscle relaxation, coping self-talk, problem-solving skills, exposure, and reward modules to the patient by utilizing relevant child-centered examples and stimuli. Matching core cognitive-behavioral tasks to interests and strengths of the child improves satisfaction with treatment and contributes to reductions in symptomology [37]. Rather than following a sequential manual, clinicians need to conceptualize and plan treatment around the contextual issues that influence their patients' presenting problems. Integration of various psychosocial challenges and deliberate attention to distinctive cultural norms are key aspects to practicing CBT with young immigrants.

Cultural adaptation occurs at all phases of treatment from the development, evaluation, and creation of interventions [12]. For example, clinicians working with Latino patients without knowledge of familismo—the importance of the physical and emotional closeness of the family—could damage treatment by not including multiple members of the family in their intervention [40]. In summary, cultural adaptations for immigrant youth simply entail that a clinician appropriately shape treatment to the individual—a fundamental requirement for all young patients.

Case Conceptualization

Effective case conceptualization is the mechanism by which a clinician flexibly designs treatment in a developmentally appropriate and culturally responsive manner. Case conceptualizations are fluid, dynamic, and change over time [10]. Through mutual collaboration between therapist and patient, an individualized, contextualized description of a patient's inner world and external environment is developed [10]. An effective case conceptualization is not a theoretical exercise; instead, it has practicality in promoting greater flexibility in customizing treatment that is culturally responsive and evidenced based—aspects of particular relevance in treatment with immigrant youth.

Data Needed for Case Conceptualization Clinicians develop case conceptualizations based on objective and subjective data gathered about the presenting problem. Data is gathered along a cluster of six symptom areas that include physiological factors, mood, behavioral symptoms, behavioral functioning, cognitions, and interpersonal relationships [41]. In addition, to individualize the descriptions, clinicians must gather data about patients' developmental history, cultural context, cognitive structures, and behavioral antecedents and consequences [42]. Perhaps most importantly, practitioners must consider these variables as conjointly influencing each other through a dynamic interplay.

Integral to conceptualization with immigrant youth is the careful consideration and integration of cultural context, self-identity, and levels of acculturation and assimilation [35, 43]. For instance, behavioral responses may be the consequence of cultural beliefs and norms or may be functional responses to sexism, racism, discrimination, and oppression. Knowledge of patients' experiences with power structures, privilege, oppression, marginalization, stereotyping, and prejudice are critical to painting a picture of their outer and inner worlds. Learning about patients' experiences with racially or ethnically charged teasing or bullying provides an important frame to understand the expression of particular symptoms [35, 43]. Therefore, careful consideration of cultural context and identities allows clinicians to assess responses to environmental stimuli and treatment interventions [35, 43].

Design and Function of Case Conceptualization Case conceptualization follows an inductive approach. Inferences and hypotheses are drawn from observations and data. Friedberg and McClure [10] describe the cognitive therapist as relying on interview data, assessment instruments, objective self-report measures, objective checklists, verbal reports, and clinical impressions. Friedberg et al. [43] are also quick to note that case conceptualizations, because they are inferentially based, are not "marble statues of patients....hardened in stone" but instead are "hypotheses written in sand" (p. 26). Collaborative empiricism, guided discovery, and flexibility are necessary to revise hypotheses, formulate new ones, and discard those that have been disconfirmed.

Case conceptualization is a foundation of clinical practice (e.g., [35]) because it serves a number of important functions. In fact, case conceptualization is essential to sound treatment processes when working with patients from diverse cultural, racial, and ethnic backgrounds [10, 44, 45]. Advantages of case conceptualization include the promotion of patient engagement, normalizing presenting issues, validation of patients' experiences, simplification of more complex and numerous problems, identification of strengths, and the promotion of resiliency [41]. Finally, case conceptualization facilitates a transdiagnostic approach to treatment thereby allowing a clinician to individualize therapy by selecting tools from evidenced-based treatments that will facilitate change, alleviate distress, and provide for efficacious treatment.

Case Study

Carolina is a 16-year-old girl who immigrated from El Salvador at age six with her father. Since then, several aunts, uncles, and cousins have joined them, but her grandmother and a number of other cousins remain in El Salvador. Carolina speaks English fluently and appears highly acculturated; her father is able to communicate in English but prefers to speak Spanish. Carolina presents to treatment after being hit by a car while on her bicycle. Since the accident, Carolina is unable to ride her bike, sit in a car, or cross the street. Carolina reports feeling "very sad" that she is such a "burden" on her father and feels embarrassed that she is not getting her driver's permit like all her friends. Carolina also experiences panic attacks, which have increased in frequency since the accident. She notes trouble sleeping, feeling tired "every day," difficulty paying attention in class, and frequent headaches.

Aside from the two days she spent in the hospital after the car accident, Carolina has an unremarkable developmental and medical history. Her father reports no significant family history for medical or psychiatric problems. Carolina moved to the USA after her mother died from a brain aneurysm in El Salvador. Since that time, Carolina has been very fearful for her own, her father's, and her grandmother's health. Carolina also worries about school, friends, and getting into college. Although Carolina was raised Catholic, she eschewed religion at the onset of adolescence because she "refused to believe God would plan to take [her] mother." Carolina's father continues to invite her to church, but her youth group friends stopped calling and she feels like the church community rejected her.

Carolina's recent car accident and the unexpected loss of her mother generated perceptions of herself as unable to exert control over her environment. In her mind, her father was forced to uproot them from their home and bring them to the USA as a result of her weakness. Even now, she is unable to contribute to the family by getting her driver's license and alleviating her father's care-giving responsibilities. Her cultural identity as a Latina immigrant youth exacerbated these perceptions as she believed she must be perfect in every way to justify her father's sacrifices in moving to the USA. The void created by Carolina's decision to stop attending church represented a significant loss of spiritual and emotional support for Carolina. She no longer believes life "has a plan" as she did before and the abrupt loss of her peers reinforced the intransience of social support.

Based on the relevant information, a parsimonious provisional formulation was constructed. Carolina's early learning history involved the sudden and unexpected death of her mother, followed closely by immigration to the USA. As a result, Carolina experienced her world as filled with invisible dangers, where tragedy strikes without warning and is accompanied by dire consequences. She was, therefore, predisposed to anxious feelings and perceptions. This vulnerability led to a tendency to focus on threat-related information both internally and externally. Carolina thus interpreted physiological sensations as catastrophic, leading to panic attacks. In her environment, peers, teachers, and strangers each evoked a level of fear. The car accident served as a confirmatory experience that Carolina is, indeed, in danger at all times. The formulation that Carolina and her clinician developed to understand her distress is succinctly summarized with the following: "I am unsafe, weak, incapable, and only cause problems for the people who care about me. I am trapped in an unpredictable, volatile world that is riddled with danger and people exist to harm me or leave me." Thus, treatment targets for Carolina included relaxation skills and cognitive restructuring for catastrophic thoughts related to her safety and distortions about social relationships. Therapy concluded with numerous experiments to assess a realistic threat level.

Therapeutic Stance Variables

Collaborative Empiricism Collaborative empiricism is an essential therapeutic stance in CBT. It is a data-driven process whereby the clinician and patient work together toward treatment goals. For example, the patient and therapist gather information about the patient's thoughts and design experiments to systematically test these thoughts [10, 46]]. Rather than being prescriptive, the clinician assumes a curious approach in which "let's find out" is a key phrase [47, 48]. The goal of collaborative empiricism is not to directly dispute a patient's thoughts but rather to replace certainty with doubt [47]. Collaborative empiricism instills a greater sense of control over the treatment process. In fact, collaboration is the variable that explains the most variance in the therapeutic relationship and is positively associated with patient engagement in treatment tasks and understanding of treatment goals [49–51]. Although collaborative empiricism is a cornerstone of CBT with any population, it is particularly critical with youth because young people are frequently in a position of low power. Ultimately, this collaborative process allows for a gradual increase in autonomy. By the end of care, the patient is able to independently implement CBT techniques without the therapist, thereby maintaining treatment progress and fostering relapse prevention.

Transparency Transparency in CBT highlights the importance of clinicians working openly and honestly with young patients. There is necessarily a difference in power between a clinician and patient, and this difference is even more profound when working with youth [52]. A transparent clinician directly and explicitly addresses power and privilege with patients. Furthermore, transparency serves to decrease the mysteriousness of the therapeutic process [52]. In other words, the clinician does not act as an omnipotent expert, but rather is forthcoming about case conceptualization, assessment, and treatment planning using clear language. Transparency allows for genuine informed consent and facilitates the development of a candid therapeutic alliance [52].

Guided Discovery Guided discovery is another critical therapeutic stance variable in CBT for youth. Guided discovery is the process by which the clinician adopts a curious and nonjudgmental clinical position to assist patients in drawing their own conclusions [10, 46]. Guided discovery occurs through the use of the Socratic method, which relies upon the systematic use of questions, inductive reasoning, identification of patterns, fostering of cognitive dissonance, and changing perspectives [53]. Therapists carefully design questions that are goal directed and draw patients' attention to maladaptive patterns and overgeneralizations [53]. For example, rather than telling patients which facts will or will not support a specific belief, the therapist uses strategically chosen questions to allow patients to discover these truths themselves. As a result, patients are more willing to accept these conclusions than if the clinician provided them directly [10].

Session Structure

Session structure is a fundamental aspect of practicing competent CBT. Structured sessions allow treatment to address maladaptive behaviors in a methodical manner [9, 10]. A proper session of CBT includes these essential steps: (1) a mood check-in, (2) setting the agenda for the session, (3) processing the information from session,

(4) creating homework assignments with the patient, and (5) summarizing the session and eliciting feedback from the patient [9, 10]. As with all components of CBT, it is important to fit the patient's conceptualization and presenting problems [9].

Mood Check-In Sessions begin with a mood check-in. For clinicians working with younger children, drawing a face depicting their mood will suffice; whereas, for older children verbal reports and objective measures are given in order to make this process more enjoyable for youth [52]. Target-monitoring questionnaires completed by the child such as the SCARED [54], the CDI-2 [55], and the SNAP IV [56] supply the therapist with objective data based on scores. The mood check-in supplies the clinician with a baseline of patients' emotional state and assists young patients with the enhancement of emotional competence through verbalization of their feelings [10].

Agenda Setting Setting the agenda helps the therapist to prioritize issues to be discussed during the session. Agenda setting is a collaborative effort in CBT. The agenda consists of both the practitioner's planned objectives and topics solicited from the patient [57]. Clinicians must remain mindful of their case conceptualization rather than responding in a knee-jerk fashion to the patient's most recent distressing incident [35]. For youths who have many topics they want to address, it is critical for the clinician to model the importance of prioritizing goals [10]. Agenda setting is a vital element in guiding therapy.

Session Content and Process Processing consists of various therapeutic techniques including empathy, Socratic questioning, problem-solving, and behavioral experiments [10]. It is important for clinicians to apply these techniques and procedures in the context of patients' negative affective arousal [58, 59]. Friedberg and McClure [10] note that a CBT clinician must master the balance between structure, process, and content. Therapeutic structure consists of the tasks rooted in a CBT framework. Thought records, games, and homework are enduring aspects of treatment that are maintained over the course of therapy [58]. Structural components evoke the content. Thoughts, feelings, and behaviors generated by the session activities are examples of therapeutic content. Last, the therapeutic process reflects a child's psychological presence in therapy. The manner in which the child completes the tasks within therapy, responds to the clinician's questions, and solves problems can showcase this presence. Derived from the content of the session, the next essential step in CBT is to create a homework assignment with the patient.

Homework Homework is vital to maintaining the progression of therapy. Practicing new skills outside of the therapy session is crucial to achieving therapeutic change [57]. CBT requires real-world implementation that is relevant to what the patient experiences in everyday life [57]. A sound homework assignment has a rationale and is explicitly related to the patient's problems [9]. Homework assignments are determined via an active collaboration between the therapist and child [10]. Tracking homework completion supplies the therapist and patient with objective metrics to evaluate levels of progress [52]. If a homework assignment is deemed unhelpful by the patient, changes are made using the gathered empirical data. Rather than viewing homework incompletion as therapeutic noncompliance, a CBT therapist examines the potential barriers to completion of the task and collaboratively devises a more attainable exercise [57]. After the homework is agreed upon, the patient is given the opportunity to provide feedback on the session.

Session Summary and Feedback The session summary is a vital aspect of therapy. It is an opportunity to reinforce the most important aspects of that session [9]. Beck [9] recommends leaving 5–10 min at the end of each appointment to sufficiently review the session and collect feedback. With younger children, session summaries can take the form of a game in which the child teaches the parents what was accomplished in session [57]. During this process, the therapists inquire what the patient found to be helpful and what was less helpful during the session [10]. It is beneficial to vary the questions used to elicit feedback, as children tend to experience difficulties providing feedback to adults in positions of authority [10, 52]. The clinician's request for feedback from the patient prevents unspoken negative feelings from festering as the patient is encouraged to identify any dissatisfaction with the session [10]. Therapists need not fear the feedback they receive from their patients. Providing young patients the time to give feedback on their treatment strengthens the therapeutic alliance and assists the therapeutic process [9].

Modular CBT

Definition of Modular CBT

Modular treatments evolved out of the discovery that many evidence-based interventions shared more commonalities than differences [59]. By distilling the multitude of intervention programs down to critical elements, core strategies were arranged into "modules" [52, 60, 61] (see Table 1). Clinicians can select and arrange components into an individualized treatment plan. In other words, rather than following a session-by-session manual, modularity allows clinicians to flexibly adapt to an individual patient's needs by responding to crises that arise during treatment, changes in symptom presentation, and complex comorbidity [61]. Thus, modular CBT specifically integrates clinician judgment into the protocol [61]. This

Table 1 Components of modular CBT

Module	Treatment target
Psychoeducation	Increase understanding of therapy and psychopathology
Target monitoring	Enhance awareness of concrete manifestations of psychopathology Gather data to use in later modules
Basic behavioral task	Acquisition of skills to change overt behaviors
Cognitive restructuring	Reduce cognitive distortions and improve mental flexibility
Exposures	Experiential learning to apply skills gained in situations that evoke negative affect

flexibility also allows clinicians to integrate culture-specific adaptations into treatment while maintaining the elements that are critical mechanisms of change.

Cutting-edge research supports the efficacy of modular approaches with youth. Weisz and Chorpita [61] developed the Modular Approach to Therapy for Children with Anxiety, Depression, Trauma or Conduct Problems (MATCH-ADTC), a comprehensive treatment protocol that allows clinicians to target up to four major symptoms clusters in one package. For example, psychoeducation, self-monitoring, and exposure are core procedures for anxiety, while active ignoring and contingency contracting may be implemented to address disruptive behavior. Instead of addressing the disorders distinctly, modular CBT presents clinicians with a road map of evidence-based elements that can be integrated to simultaneously target the observed deficits [61].

Termed *relevance mapping*, the "mix-and-match" approach combines the strengths of empirically supported treatments with culturally sensitive care [32, 62]. Relevance mapping software takes into account a youth's age, gender, ethnicity, and presenting problem to determine the most applicable interventions as determined by research [62]. By using this approach, more youth are able to be treated more effectively [62].

Importantly, emerging literature supports that modular treatment is associated with faster improvement than manualized CBT or usual care [63]. Lyon and colleagues [32] review the ways in which clinicians easily integrate cultural variations using modular CBT, highlighting the efficiency of this framework that delivers the necessary tools to treat a broad range of youth.

Psychoeducation

Psychoeducation involves orienting youth and their parents to the treatment process. This includes providing information about the child's presenting problem and discussing what to expect from the treatment approach [64]. Introducing families to the therapy process is particularly important with immigrant youth, whose families may not be familiar with psychotherapy. Explaining what to expect, addressing misconceptions, and providing information about the young patient's symptoms facilitates motivation and investment in treatment [58]. Skillful psychoeducation contributes to engagement in treatment. Cultural variables are easily integrated into this module.

For example, using a culturally and individually relevant metaphor to explain treatment fosters understanding and builds the therapeutic relationship. With an adolescent Mexican-American male who was a fan of sports, depression was once described as being like an injured soccer player, and treatment involves strategies to get the athlete back on the field. Culturally relevant analogies can also be used in describing the structure of cognitive-behavioral treatment.

With youth, it is particularly important that clinicians are creative in the implementation of psychoeducation. For example, multimedia including picture books, movies, songs, pamphlets, websites, and TV shows can be employed to communicate critical information [52]. Practitioners should strive to provide information in a variety of different mediums to facilitate understanding and meet the needs of each unique family. For example, parents can be given printed material from websites (e.g., www.aboutourkids.com, www.effectivechildtherapy.com, www.aacap.org, www.nimh.org), and clinicians can read a picture book with young children (e.g., *What to Do When You Worry Too Much* [65]). Psychoeducational material should be presented in the preferred language of parent and child.

Target Monitoring

Target monitoring is the data collection phase of treatment and serves to both increase awareness and establish a baseline of symptoms. Patients and/or parents are asked to track thoughts, feelings, behaviors, and physiological sensations—essentially, patients gather information relevant to their presenting problem [64]. Thought records are one example of a method for monitoring automatic thoughts, situations that elicit particular beliefs, and patterns of cognitive distortions [64]. Target-monitoring techniques can and should be adapted to the patient's age, cultural background, interests, etc. For example, young children respond well to filling in faces with expressions or coloring in a thermometer to reflect the intensity of their emotions; adolescents may simply report intensity on a scale from 0 to 10. Cultural adaptations can easily be integrated into this module as well. For example, a young Chinese patient may experience her anxiety primarily as somatic symptoms such as stomachache, numbness, tingling, and racing heart. As a result, monitoring somatic symptoms and physiological arousal using culture-specific language (e.g., blockages of Xi) rather than asking her to rate her anxiety will make this module more relevant.

Clinicians can also utilize self-report measures such as the Children's Depression Inventory (CDI-2 [55]) and Screen for Child Anxiety Related Emotional Disorders (SCARED) [54]. The CDI-2 is available in English and Spanish, and the SCARED is available in Arabic, Chinese, English, French, German, Italian, Portuguese, and Spanish. These measures allow young patients and families to monitor symptoms over time using objective assessment.

Target monitoring also facilitates functional analysis of problem behaviors by identifying antecedents and consequences [38]. Furthermore, monitoring emotional intensity in response to feared situations enables patients and clinicians to collaboratively develop a hierarchy of feared stimuli for graduated exposure [61, 66]. In short, target monitoring provides essential data that guides later phases of treatment.

Basic Behavioral Tasks

Basic behavioral tasks relevant to a patient's presentation are identified by reviewing data collected from the target-monitoring module. Techniques are designed from classical conditioning, operant conditioning, and social learning theory. Behavioral procedures aim to change overt actions. Through practice of these activities, patients acquire new tools to more effectively cope with distress and change action tendencies associated with heightened emotional arousal [67, 68]. Basic behavioral tasks are particularly relevant to many immigrant youth as somatic symptoms are often predominant with these patients [69, 70].

For example, the ideal behavioral tasks for a child who reports significant anxiety marked by autonomic hyperarousal and somatic complaints include relaxation techniques. Diaphragmatic breathing or progressive muscle relaxation teaches the patient to interrupt the pattern of physiological hyperarousal [58]. Activities for youth combating depression include pleasant activities scheduling or behavioral activation to mitigate the lethargy induced by depression. These interventions augment sources of positive reinforcement and improve mood [58]. Social skills training, habit reversal training, contingency contracts, and implementation of reward systems are other available procedures [52, 60, 71]. Basic behavioral tasks actively and explicitly teach the child that he/she is able to exert some control over distressful experiences. Skills gained in this module instill hope, motivate patients to progress in treatment, and pave the way for future interventions. Two clinical examples of the way behavioral tasks were designed to attend to important cultural factors with immigrant patients and their families are described.

Case Study 1

Dakila (6) and Bayani (7) immigrated to the USA with their parents from the Philippines for their father's work when they were 4 and 5. The family presented to treatment for help with sibling conflict and behavioral outbursts that onset the year following their immigration to the USA when the boys were 4 and 5. The parents were hesitant to implement behavior charts because they felt overwhelmed with the number of behaviors that they hoped to change. Additionally, both parents worked two jobs and were concerned that the system would be inconsistent between caregivers (mother, father, aunt). They were also unwilling to "reward bad behavior," feeling like the boys "should" get along because they were family. The clinician suggested that in place of devising individual contingency contracts, the boys would have a joint reward system. The mother used a jar and added marbles to the jar each time the boys played nicely together, cooperated on chores, followed instructions, and executed other desired behaviors. When the jar was full, the boys earned a pizza night, a trip to the movies, or a picnic in the park. The parents were willing to provide family-oriented incentives, and the joint system was more manageable for the parents' busy schedules. By tailoring the behavioral tasks to fit the family's cultural values and their specific needs, the family was more engaged, and the intervention was highly successful.

Case Study 2

Nico (13) emigrated from Sudan with his 19-year-old sister and 24-year-old aunt after being granted political asylum in the USA. He developed school refusal in the year following immigration. The school was much larger and more chaotic than the academic environment he experienced in Sudan; Nico also hated the loud bells that rang often throughout the day. He endorsed substantial physiological hyperarousal upon arriving on school grounds and hated the way his skin "crawled." Nico spoke often about his desire to be in a "peaceful" place and reported that the school was so aversive because it was the "opposite" of peace. When training Nico in breathing exercises, the clinician likened the activity to "breathing in peace, and breathing out chaos." Pairing Nico's desire for peace with the behavioral intervention gave him a concrete understanding of how the exercise helped him to achieve his goals.

Cognitive Restructuring

Cognitive restructuring interventions target patients' thought content and thought processes. Youth learn to reduce cognitive distortions and train their minds to think more flexibly [58, 60, 66]. Cognitive interventions include problem-solving, reattribution, decatastrophizing, test of evidence, and self-instruction [52, 72]. The use of metaphors related to concrete ideas or the youth's interests heightens the patient's experience of cognitive interventions [64, 73].

Case Study 3

Jesper, a 9-year-old male who emigrated from Denmark with his parents within the past year, presented to therapy for generalized anxiety: Jesper's favorite thing to do was to watch sports on TV with his father. He especially loved that they could pause and rewind the game to see if the referee made a good call. Jesper and his therapist talked about how sometimes when he took time to gather more evidence, like watching replays, Jesper changed his mind. He drew a remote control and in sessions the therapist encouraged Jesper to "pause" his thoughts, "rewind" to look for evidence that either supported or refuted his beliefs, and use "slow motion" to slow down his thinking. Jesper's parents were especially pleased with the remote control exercise as they related easily to the concepts and even gave him a broken TV remote to use at home. Thus, the salience of this metaphor facilitated the use of cognitive coping skills, propelling therapy forward.

Case Study 4

Asuka, a 14-year-old Japanese girl, immigrated to the USA with her parents, brother, and grandparents when she was 10. Asuka was diagnosed with OCD and displayed contamination fears related to "sharing air" with people; she could not talk to others unless she stood several feet away to ensure she breathed "fresh" air. This dramatically interfered with her ability to develop a social support system despite the fact she found a group of girls who shared her passions for anime and manga—animated adventures in video and graphic novel formats. When she reached the cognitive restructuring module, her therapist suggested that she make her own manga to chronicle her "battles" against the OCD. Asuka delighted in the exercise and created extraordinary pages illustrating her cognitive contests against the OCD villain living in her mind. Not only did this exercise make cognitive interventions literally come alive for Asuka, it also established a way for her to open communication with her friends.

Exposures

The final module is *exposures*, the zenith of CBT. While each previous segment substantially contributes to young patients' treatment, the exposures module presents patients with the opportunity to synthesize the gains they have made thus far. The ultimate experiential learning, young patients engage in exposures to emotionally evocative stimuli then apply coping skills learned throughout therapy. These interventions transform patients' action tendencies and eliminate maladaptive behavior patterns.

Founded on the social learning theory, concepts of performance attainment and mastery are the mechanisms through which distress is relieved [58, 74]. Effective exposures must take place in the context of emotional arousal so that patients truly learn how to utilize coping skills in the face of their ultimate stressors [73–75]. Clinicians collaboratively devise exercises where patients face challenging situations identified in the hierarchy from the target-monitoring module [73]. Exercises begin with situations that elicit a moderate level of discomfort; patients confront the experiences and employ adaptive strategies to either reduce distress or tolerate the uneasiness. If the exposure is executed properly, patients' fear of the stimulus is diminished. In this fashion, patients "climb their ladders" as they move through situations ranked as increasingly upsetting. Termination of care is indicated once patients leap these hurdles.

Case Study 5

Mitra, age 11, was an Iranian; she and her parents left Iran when she was 3 and moved in with an aunt, uncle, and four cousins in the USA. Her parents brought her to therapy for treatment of anger outbursts that occurred solely in the context of school. Upon intake, Mitra had been suspended twice for fighting. Her parents were so perplexed by her behavior; they were considering sending her back to live with family in Iran. Therapy revealed that Mitra was lashing out at peers physically in response to ethnically charged teasing. Mitra lacked complex language skills to be able to "fight back" with her words. Mitra created a hierarchy specific to the behaviors of her peers that "made her explode." The lower-rated behaviors included people staring at her, pointing, and whispering and then climbed to name-calling and physical contact (e.g., pushing her).

After learning skills to use when she "got hot," Mitra and her therapist went out into the waiting room wearing different props to attract people's stares. Mitra noted that she did not feel as angry when adults looked at her as she did when other youth did. Therefore, to make the exercise more relevant, Mitra and her therapist went to sit in a pediatrician's waiting room.

For the final step, Mitra and the therapist went into a crowded coffee shop close to the clinic to practice how to remain calm when others bumped into her. When they first began this step, Mitra's father came to the coffee shop with them. Mitra realized that she felt safe with her father near, stating "he will always take care of me." Thus, they pursued further practice with no parent nearby. Because the therapist attended closely to the level of emotional activation evoked by the interventions, Mitra was able to generalize her learning to the school environment and finished the academic year without another fight.

Case Study 6

Tammy (15) was born in the USA but lived in Vietnam with her mother from the ages of 7 to 11 to care for her dying grandfather. During that time, her father and older brother stayed in the USA. She presented to treatment for restricted eating behaviors. Tammy played varsity basketball; she was smaller than her teammates but fast and very skilled. She told her therapist that she feels "short and fat" and all her friends are "tall and thin." She also reported that she feels "out of place" with her friends and that her parents "just don't get it." Tammy stopped eating meals at school, refrains from eating in public, and recently fainted during basketball practice. When she reached the exposure module of treatment, she and her therapist made plans to conquer the steps on her ladder: sitting in an eating establishment with food on her plate, eating something "unhealthy" in front of others, ordering food at a restaurant, and eating with friends.

A significant amount of Tammy's distress emerged from the fact that she perceived implicit scrutiny from friends who were "so different." Tammy's therapist was a young female Caucasian; thus, the therapeutic relationship itself presented opportunities for exposure. Tammy and her therapist conducted all exposure steps in a café. For Tammy's final exposure, she invited her basketball team to her house for a pizza party. By actively engaging in experiential learning, patients learn firsthand that their coping tools work, and they are able to tolerate situations that previously seemed unbearable [58].

Conclusion

Disney proclaims, "A smile means friendship to everyone" in their song "It's a Small World" [76]. CBT is no different as the modifications needed to make CBT relevant to immigrant youth are no more than those a proficient CBT clinician would construct to match a patient of any age or background. Some question whether CBT thoroughly addresses the complex concerns of immigrant youth; these doubts reflect insufficient grasp of the execution of skillful CBT. The flexibility inherent in the modular cognitive-behavioral model mandates careful attention to all cultural identities [32, 77]. If faced with challenges such as difficulty with verbal techniques or a language barrier, clinicians may adapt interventions to use play or nonverbal techniques (e.g., art/drawing). To augment generalization of skills, therapists can utilize family members, community supports, and/or teachers as indicated by the needs of the immigrant patient. Each of these represents a faithful alteration to treatment as the original mechanisms of change are maintained; the mode of delivery is tailored to the specific youth's needs.

As discussed throughout the chapter, modifications needed for work with immigrant youth are simple adjustments in content and area of focus, not to the model or mechanisms of change [12, 31]. Psychosocial factors specific to immigrant youth are readily addressed [28, 32], for example, including influential people in treatment when appropriate (e.g., family, teachers, community leaders), ensuring homework is achievable given patient's circumstances, and adding interventions to the modules that directly address ways to manage perceived discrimination. Furthermore, while there is limited evidence in support of the effectiveness of CBT with a wide range of immigrant youth, there is a total absence of data to suggest CBT impacts young immigrants adversely.

CBT is a theoretically sound, empirically supported, and easily adaptable treatment. The innovative design of modular CBT further enhances the benefits young patients gain from a therapy that is intimately tailored to fit their specific presenting problems. In order to deliver this efficacious treatment to immigrant youth, however, clinicians must practice faithful CBT. This chapter outlines the essential elements of CBT, attending to both content and process factors. Additionally, the chapter illustrates each component of treatment in the context of a clinical experience with a young immigrant patient.

Clinicians treating immigrant youth must develop a robust case conceptualization to address the layered complexities often present in young immigrant patients. The use of CBT with immigrant youth in particular allows for clinicians to appropriately adapt exercises to idiosyncratic symptom presentation, interests, and psychosocial contexts. From that formulation, clinicians must fashion treatment to specifically target the maintaining factors of the patient's distress. When therapy is accurately guided by a precise conceptualization, clinicians fluidly move from module to module as they target discrete behavioral excesses and deficits evidenced by youth. Using these skills, clinicians will provide immigrant youth with the much-needed support they seek in this "small, small world."

References

1. Huey SJ, Tilley JL, Jones EO, Smith CA. The contribution of cultural competence to evidence-based care for ethnically diverse populations. Annu Rev Clin Psychol. 2014;10:305–38. doi:10.1146/annurev-clinpsy-032813-153729.
2. Kataoka SH, Stein BD, Jaycox LH, Wong M, Escudero P, Tu W, et al. A school-based mental health program for traumatized Latino immigrant children. J Am Acad Child Adolesc Psychiatry. 2003;42(3):311–8.
3. Nicolas G, Arntz DL, Hirsch B, Schmiedigen A. Cultural adaptation of a group treatment for Haitian American adolescents. Prof Psychol Res Pr. 2009;40(4):378–84.
4. Stein BD, Jaycox LH, Kataoka SH, Wong M, Tu W, Elliott MN, et al. A mental health intervention for school children exposed to violence: a randomized controlled trial. JAMA. 2003;290(5):603–11. doi:10.1001/jama.290.5.603.
5. Huey Jr SJ, Polo AJ. Evidence-based psychosocial treatments for ethnic minority youth. J Clin Child Adolesc Psychol. 2008;37(1):262–301.
6. Pumariega AJ, Rothe E. Leaving no children or families outside: the challenges of immigration. Am J Orthopsychiatry. 2010;80(4):505–15.
7. Rettger JP, Kletter H, Carrion V. Trauma and acculturative stress. In: Patel S, Reicherter D, editors. Psychotherapy for immigrant youth. New York: Springer; 2015.
8. Ngo V, Langley A, Kataoka SH, Nadeem E, Escudero P, Stein BD. Providing evidence-based practice to ethnically diverse youths: Examples from the Cognitive Behavioral Intervention for Trauma in Schools (CBITS) program. J Am Acad Child Adolesc Psychiatry. 2008;47(8):858–62.
9. Beck JS. Cognitive behavior therapy: basics and beyond. 2nd ed. Guilford: New York, NY; 2011.
10. Friedberg RD, McClure JM. Clinical practice of cognitive therapy with children and adolescents: the nuts and bolts. 2nd ed. Guilford: New York, NY; 2015.
11. Benish SG, Quintana S, Wampold BE. Culturally adapted psychotherapy and the legitimacy of myth: a direct comparison meta-analysis. J Couns Psychol. 2011;58:279–89.
12. Cardemil EV. Cultural adaptations to empirically supported treatments: a research agenda. Sci Rev Ment Health Pract. 2010;7(2):8–21.
13. La Roche M, Christopher M. Changing paradigms from empirically supported treatments to evidenced based practice: a cultural perspective. Prof Psychol Res Pr. 2009;40:396–402.
14. Kazdin AE. Evidence-based treatment and practice: new opportunities to bridge clinical research and practice, enhance the knowledge base, and improve patient care. Am Psychol. 2008;63:146–59.
15. Kendall PC, Hudson JL, Gosch E, Flannery-Schroeder E, Suveg C. Cognitive-behavioral therapy for anxiety disordered youth: a randomized clinical trial evaluating child and family modalities. J Consult Clin Psychol. 2008;76(2):282–97. doi:10.1037/0022-006X.76.2.282.
16. Walkup JT, Albano AM, Piacentini J, Birmaher B, Compton SN, Sherrill JT, et al. Cognitive behavioral therapy, sertraline or a combination in childhood anxiety. N Engl J Med. 2008;359(26):2753–66.

17. Franklin ME, Sapyta J, Freeman JB, Khanna M, Compton SN, Almirall D, et al. Cognitive behavior therapy augmentation of pharmacotherapy in pediatric obsessive-compulsive disorder. J Am Med Assoc. 2011;306(11):1224–32.
18. March JS, Vitiello B. Clinical messages from the Treatment of Adolescents with Depression Study (TADS). Am J Psychiatr. 2009;166:1118–23.
19. Cohen JA, Deblinger E, Mannarino AP, Steer R. A multi-site, randomized controlled trial for children with abuse related PTSD symptoms. J Am Acad Child Adolesc Psychiatry. 2004;43(4):393–402.
20. Lochman JE, Powell NP, Boxmeyer CL, Jimenez-Camargo L. Cognitive-behavioral therapy for externalizing disorders in children and adolescents. Child Adolesc Psychiatr Clin N Am. 2011;20(2):305–18.
21. Eyberg SM, Nelson MM, Boggs SR. Evidence-based psychosocial treatments for children and adolescents with disruptive behavior. J Clin Child Adolesc Psychol. 2008;37(1):215–37. doi:10.1080/15374410701820117.
22. Wood JJ, Drahota A, Sze K, Har K, Chiu A, Langer DA. Cognitive behavioral therapy for anxiety in children with autism spectrum disorders: a randomized, controlled trial. J Child Psychol Psychiatry. 2009;50(3):224–34. doi:10.1111/j.1469-7610.2008.01948.x.
23. Sofronoff K, Attwood T, Hinton S. A randomised controlled trial of a CBT intervention for anxiety in children with Asperger syndrome. J Child Psychol Psychiatry. 2005;46(11):1152–60. doi:10.1111/j.1469-7610.2005.00411.x.
24. White SW, Ollendick T, Albano AM, Oswald D, Johnson C, Southam-Gerow MA, et al. Randomized controlled trial: Multimodal Anxiety and Social Skill Intervention for adolescents with autism spectrum disorder. J Autism Dev Disord. 2013;43(2):382–94. doi:10.1007/s10803-012-1577-x.
25. Waldron HB, Turner CW. Evidence based psychosocial treatments for adolescent substance abuse. J Clin Child Adolesc Psychol. 2008;37(1):238–61. doi:10.1080/15374410701820133.
26. Keel PK, Haedt A. Evidence-based psychosocial treatments for eating problems and eating disorders. J Clin Child Adolesc Psychol. 2008;37(1):39–61. doi:10.1080/15374410701817832.
27. Beehler S, Birman D, Campbell R. The effectiveness of cultural adjustment and trauma services (CATS): generating practice-based evidence on a comprehensive, school-based mental health intervention for immigrant youth. Am J Community Psychol. 2012;50(1–2):155–68.
28. Dattilio FM, Bahadur M. Cognitive behavioral therapy with an East Indian family. Contemp Fam Ther. 2005;27(3):367–82.
29. Sandil R. Cognitive behavioral therapy for adolescent depression: Implications for Asian immigrants to the United States of America. J Child Adolesc Ment Health. 2006;18(1):27–32.
30. Patel SG, Tabb KM, Strambler MJ, Eltareb F. Newcomer immigrant adolescents and ambiguous discrimination the role of cognitive appraisal. J Adolesc Res. 2015;30(1):7–30.
31. Hays PA. Integrating evidence-based practice, cognitive-behavior therapy, and multicultural therapy: ten steps for culturally competent practice. Prof Psychol Res Pr. 2009;40(4):354–60.
32. Lyon AR, Lau AS, McCauley E, Vander Stoep A, Chorpita BF. A case for modular design: implications for implementing evidence-based interventions with culturally diverse youth. Prof Psychol Res Pr. 2014;45(1):57.
33. Kendall PC, Beidas RS. Smoothing the trail for dissemination of evidence-based practices for youth: flexibility within fidelity. Prof Psychol Res Pr. 2007;38(1):13–20. doi:10.1037/0735-7028.38.1.13.
34. Kataoka S, Novins DK, DeCarlo Santiago C. The practice of evidence-based treatments in ethnic minority youth. Child Adolesc Psychiatr Clin N Am. 2010;19(4):775–89.
35. Friedberg RD, Gorman AA, Beidel DC. Training psychologists for cognitive-behavioral therapy in the raw world: A rubric for supervisors. Behav Modif. 2009;33(1):104–23. doi:10.1177/0145445508322609.
36. Beidas RS, Koerner K, Wiengardt KR, Kendall PC. Training research: practical recommendations for maximum impact. Admin Pol Ment Health. 2011;38(4):223–37.

37. Kendall PC, Gosch E, Furr JM, Sood E. Flexibility within fidelity. J Am Acad Child Adolesc Psychiatry. 2008;47(9):987–93. doi:10.1097/CHI.0b013e31817eed2f.
38. Chorpita BF, Taylor AA, Francis SE, Moffitt C, Austin AA. Efficacy of modular cognitive behavior therapy for childhood anxiety disorders. Behav Ther. 2004;35(2):263–87. doi:10.1016/S0005-7894(04)80039-X.
39. Kendall PC, Hedtke K. Cognitive-behavioral therapy for anxious children: therapist manual. 3rd ed. Ardmore, PA: Workbook Publishing; 2006.
40. Bernal G, Cumba-Aviles E, Saez-Santiago E. Cultural and relational processes in depressed Latino adolescents. In: Beach SRH, Wamboldt MZ, Kaslow NJ, Heyman RE, Reiss D, editors. Relational processes and DSM-V: neuroscience, assessment, prevention and treatment. Washington, DC: American Psychiatric Association; 2006. p. 221–4.
41. Kuyken W, Padesky CA, Dudley R. Collaborative case conceptualization: working effectively with clients in cognitive-behavioral therapy. Guilford: New York, NY; 2008.
42. Pearl AM, Mahr F, Friedberg RD. Supervising child psychiatry fellows in cognitive behavioral therapy: crucibles and choices. J Cogn Psychother. 2013;27(1):61–71.
43. Friedberg RD, Gorman AA, Wilt LH, Biuckians A, Murray M. Cognitive behavioral therapy for the busy child psychiatrist and other mental health professionals: rubrics and rudiments. New York, NY: Routledge; 2011.
44. Macneil CA, Hasty MK, Conus P, Berk M. Is diagnosis enough to guide interventions in mental health? Using case formulation in clinical practice. BMC Med. 2012;10(1):111–3.
45. Persons JB. Cognitive therapy in practice: a case formulation approach. New York: Norton; 1989. p. 109–18.
46. Overholser JC. Collaborative empiricism, guided discovery, and the Socratic method: core processes for effective cognitive therapy. Clin Psychol Sci Pract. 2011;18(1):62–6.
47. Padesky CA, Greenberger D. Clinician's guide to mind over mood. Guilford: New York, NY; 1995.
48. Southam-Gerow MA. Emotion regulation in children and adolescents: a practitioner's guide. Guilford: New York, NY; 2013.
49. Creed TA, Kendall PC. Therapist alliance-building behavior within a cognitive-behavioral treatment for anxiety in youth. J Consult Clin Psychol. 2005;73(3):498–505. doi:10.1037/0022-006X.73.3.498.
50. Kingery JN, Roblek TL, Suveg C, Grover RL, Sherrill JT, Bergman RL. They're not just "little adults": developmental considerations for implementing cognitive-behavioral therapy with anxious youth. J Cogn Psychother. 2006;20(3):263–73. doi:10.1891/088983906780644037.
51. Podell JL, Kendall PC, Gosch EA, Compton SN, March JS, Albano A-M, et al. Therapist factors and outcomes in CBT for anxiety in youth. Prof Psychol Res Pr. 2013;44(2):89–98. doi:10.1037/a0031700.
52. Friedberg RD, Brelsford GM. Core principles in cognitive therapy with youth. Child Adolesc Psychiatr Clin N Am. 2011;20(2):369–78. doi:10.1016/j.chc.2011.01.009.
53. Overholser JC. Psychotherapy according to the Socratic method: integrating ancient philosophy with contemporary cognitive therapy. J Cogn Psychother. 2010;24(4):354–63. doi:10.1891/0889-8391.24.4.354.
54. Birmaher B, Khetarpal S, Brent D, Cully M, Balach L, Kaufman J, et al. The screen for child anxiety related emotional disorders (SCARED): scale construction and psychometric characteristics. J Am Acad Child Adolesc Psychiatry. 1997;36(4):545–53.
55. Kovacs M. The children's depression inventory: manual. Multi-Health Systems: North Tonawanda, NY; 1992.
56. Swanson JM. SNAP-IV scale. Irvine, CA: University of California Child Development Center; 1995.
57. Bearman SK, Weisz JR. Cognitive behavioral therapy for children and adolescents: an introduction. In: Szigethy E, Weisz JR, Findling RI, editors. CBT for children and adolescents. Washington, DC: American Psychiatric Publishing; 2012. p. 1–28.
58. Friedberg RD, McClure JM, Garcia JH. Cognitive therapy techniques for children and adolescents: tools for enhancing practice. Guilford: New York, NY; 2009.

59. Wilamowska Z, Thompson-Hollands J, Fairholme C, et al. Conceptual background, development and preliminary data from the unified protocol for transdiagnostic treatment of emotional disorders. Depress Anxiety. 2010;27(10):882–90.
60. Chorpita BF. Modular cognitive-behavioral therapy for childhood anxiety disorders. (J. Persons, Ed.). Guilford: New York, NY; 2007.
61. Weisz JR, Chorpita BF. "Mod Squad" for youth psychotherapy. In: Kendall PC, editor. Child and adolescent therapy. New York, NY: Guilford; 2012. p. 379–96.
62. Chorpita BF, Bernstein A, Daleiden EL. Empirically guided coordination of multiple evidence-based treatments: an illustration of relevance mapping in children's mental health services. J Consult Clin Psychol. 2011;79(4):470–80.
63. Weisz JR, Chorpita BF, Palinkas LA, Schoenwald SK, Miranda J, Bearman SK, et al. Testing standard and modular designs for psychotherapy treating depression, anxiety, and conduct problems in youth: a randomized effectiveness trial. Arch Gen Psychiatry. 2012;69(3):274–82. doi:10.1001/archgenpsychiatry.2011.147.
64. Friedberg RD, Gorman AA. Integrating psychotherapeutic processes with cognitive behavioral procedures. J Contemp Psychother. 2007;37(3):185–93. doi:10.1007/s10879-007-9053-1.
65. Huebner D. What to do when you worry too much: a kid's guide to overcoming anxiety. Washington, DC: Magination Press; 2005.
66. Kendall PC. Child and adolescent therapy. Guilford: New York, NY; 2006.
67. Ehrenreich JT, Goldstein CM, Wright LR, Barlow DH. Development of a unified protocol for the treatment of emotional disorders in youth. Child Fam Behav Ther. 2009;31(1):20–37. doi:10.1080/07317100802701228.
68. Chorpita BF. Modular cognitive-behavioral therapy for childhood anxiety disorders. Guilford: New York, NY; 2007.
69. Anderson ER, Mayes LC. Race/ethnicity and internalizing disorders in youth: a review. Clin Psychol Rev. 2010;30(3):338–48.
70. Kirmayer LJ, Narasiah L, Munoz M, Rashid M, Ryder AG, Guzder J, et al. Common mental health problems in immigrants and refugees: general approach in primary care. Can Med Assoc J. 2011;183(12):E959–67.
71. Kendall PC, Morris RJ. Child therapy: issues and recommendations. J Consult Clin Psychol. 1991;59(6):777–84. Retrieved from http://www.ncbi.nlm.nih.gov/pubmed/1774363.
72. Sburlati ES, Schniering CA, Lyneham HJ, Rapee RM. A model of therapist competencies for the empirically supported cognitive behavioral treatment of child and adolescent anxiety and depressive disorders. Clin Child Fam Psychol Rev. 2011;14(1):89–109. doi:10.1007/s10567-011-0083-6.
73. Peterman JS, Read KL, Wei C, Kendall PC. The art of exposure: putting science into practice. Cogn Behav Pract. 2014. doi:10.1016/j.cbpra.2014.02.003.
74. Barlow DH, Allen LB, Choate ML. Toward a unified treatment for emotional disorders. Behav Ther. 2004;35(2):205–30. doi:10.1016/S0005-7894(04)80036-4.
75. Kendall PC, Robin JA, Hedtke KA, Suveg C, Flannery-Shroeder E, Gosch E. Considering CBT with anxious youth? Think exposures Cogn Behav Pract. 2005;12:136–50.
76. Sherman RB, Sherman RM. It's a small world (after all). Anaheim, CA: Walt Disney Corporation; 1963.
77. Chorpita BF, Daleiden EL, Weisz JR. Identifying and selecting the common elements of evidence based interventions: a distillation and matching model. Ment Health Serv Res. 2005;7(1):5–20.

Family Factors: Immigrant Families and Intergenerational Considerations

Maryam Kia-Keating, Diana Capous, Linda Juang, and Guadalupe Bacio

Abstract

This chapter emphasizes the importance of paying special attention to the family context for immigrant youth. Some key considerations for immigrant families, including separation and reunification, cultural and language brokering, acculturative gaps, and family conflict, are described. Case vignettes are used to illuminate these experiences, in order to bring empirical findings to life and reflect the kinds of circumstances which practitioners may encounter in their work with immigrant families.

Keywords

Separation and reunification • Cultural and language brokering • Acculturative gaps • Family conflict • Family interventions • Prevention • Family strengths

Family Factors: Immigrant Families and Intergenerational Considerations

Family immigration histories are deeply woven into the fabric of American life, playing a central role in family and personal identities. In the USA, one in five US residents (e.g., 61.8 million individuals over age five) speaks a language other than

M. Kia-Keating, Ph.D. (✉) • D. Capous
Department of Counseling, Clinical and School Psychology, Gevirtz Graduate School of Education, University of California, Santa Barbara, Santa Barbara, CA 93106-9490, USA
e-mail: mkiakeating@education.ucsb.edu

L. Juang
Department of Education, Universität Potsdam, Potsdam, Germany

G. Bacio
Department of Psychiatry, University of California, San Diego, San Diego, CA USA

S.G. Patel, D. Reicherter (eds.), *Psychotherapy for Immigrant Youth*,
DOI 10.1007/978-3-319-24693-2_3

English at home [1, p. 1]; these include both first- and second-generation immigrants. Moreover, these statistics are higher among school-aged youth (ages 5–17) residing in particular states, such as California (44 %), Texas (35 %), and New York (30 %) [1, p. 5]. In fact, projections suggest that by the year 2020, a third of children under the age of 18 residing in the USA will be the child of a first-generation immigrant [2]. Both first-generation immigrants and their children are impacted by the multiple and interacting factors uniquely related to their families' immigration histories.

Immigrant families, including those whose migration was propelled by economic or humanitarian reasons, are often driven by the promise and hope of a better future than the one offered in their home countries, especially for the next generation. Immigration is a rather complex undertaking that presents many challenges along the way for families. Exposure to adversities begins premigration and may include unstable employment/income, limited resources, lack of educational opportunities for the children, and political conflict or upheaval [3, 4]. As discussed in greater length elsewhere in this book [5, 6], the immigration process itself can present additional difficulties depending on the path immigrants take en route to a new country. These journeys may include a range of challenges including arduous border crossings, family separations, complex legal procedures, and victimization or violence by travelers or traffickers [3]. Once immigrant families enter the host country, the reception by and settlement in the community and neighborhoods to which they arrive present a new array of challenges, such as differences in culture, language, discrimination, and adversities such as exposure to poverty [3] and community violence [7].

Theoretical Framework

When considering immigrant youth specifically, bioecological theory argues that the experiences and opportunities afforded by interactions between immigrant youth and their families, peers, schools, and communities influence their future developmental trajectories [8]. An integrated model creates a more holistic framework by taking into account the interconnectedness among the ecological systems, risk, protection, and assets [9, 10]. An ecological transactional model focuses on interactions and transactions that impact development overtime through a reciprocal process of an individual shaping and being shaped by the various contexts in which he/she lives. Risk factors increase the likelihood of the onset or maintenance of a problem state or pathology [11, 12], while protective factors function as moderators, acting as a buffer to negative outcomes [13, 14]. Finally, assets or promotive factors, including internal and external strengths within an individual's social ecology, are those that directly lead to positive and healthy outcomes [14, 15]. All three types of factors exist within immigrants' social ecologies. Successful prevention and intervention efforts underscore and capitalize on strengths and resilience, in the context of the unique challenges faced by immigrant families [16]. An approach that integrates various ecologies allows practitioners and researchers to gain a better understanding of the complex challenges, influences, and interactions of immigrant family dynamics.

The chapter provides an overarching look at these issues, covering the research findings to date related to the risk and protective factors for immigrant families defined in Table 1. However, clinicians are urged to follow multicultural guidelines for practice [17], to adequately take into account unique sociopolitical, historical, cultural, and other relevant issues that are more specific to particular clients' needs than the material provided here.

Families and Resettlement Stressors

Epidemiological mental health studies in the USA suggest that immigrants may have an advantage over their US-born counterparts. That is, immigrants seem to report lower rates of psychopathology compared to later US-born generations (e.g., [18, 19]). These differences have been observed in immigrant children; for example, in one study, using data from over 80,000 families participating in the National Survey of Children's Health, the prevalence of mental health conditions of immigrant children was about three times lower than Hispanic children from nonimmigrant families [20]. Some research has suggested that having immigrant parents may be a protective factor for children [21].

At the same time, some research has demonstrated that the mental health of immigrants deteriorates over time residing in the new host country (e.g., [22]). Although the research data on the mechanisms that explain this seeming decline in immigrant mental health are not conclusive, challenges posed by the immigration process have been shown to have a detrimental effect on the mental health of immigrant families. These challenges, described in further detail below, include acculturative stress, discrimination, exposure to violence, and trauma and may include fear and uncertainty related to their legal status in the host country.

Acculturative Stress

Immigrant families experience psychological strain resulting from acculturation processes to the new host environment in navigating and negotiating different cultures [6]; this experience has been termed acculturative stress [23]. Acculturative stressors include navigating a new setting where immigrant families may take a minority status for the first time, the challenges of gaining proficiency in a new language, lack of knowledge on how to access institutional resources (e.g., school, healthcare), and reestablishing social support, among others. Although there is evidence consistent with the expectation that acculturative stress should decline as immigrants adapt to the new culture and learn how to navigate it [22], it is not always the case. Acculturation can act as a sociocultural stressor in families when there is a gap between how quickly immigrant parents and their children acculturate [6]. Specifically, acculturative gaps can increase family conflict [24, 25] and

Table 1 Family-related risk and protective factors important to consider for immigrant families

	Definition/role
Risk factor	
Acculturative stress	Psychological strain resulting from stressors related to navigating a new environment including lack of knowledge about how to access resources (i.e., school, healthcare), learning a new language, and reestablishing social networks, among others
Acculturation gap	The nature and extent of the gap between the rate of acquisition of values and behaviors of the new culture between immigrant children and their parents. For some families, the acculturation gap can negatively impact to family dynamics and children's development
Acculturation-based conflict	Arguments rooted in cultural value differences between children and their parents. In contrast to everyday conflict, it tends to be viewed more negatively and can be a better predictor of adjustment for some families
Discrimination	Discrimination experiences based on children's/parents' immigration status and racial/ethnic background, among others. The impact of discrimination on immigrant families' mental health may depend on their individual cognitive appraisals. Intergenerational studies show that parents play a key role in their children's interpretation of and preparation for discrimination
Exposure to violence	Immigrant families can experience exposure to violence before, during, and post-migration. Parental mental health, including post-traumatic symptoms, is significantly related to children's vulnerabilities and psychosocial adjustment particularly among refugee and war-affected immigrants. Receiving communities where immigrant families resettle may also expose them to new forms of violence, which also negatively impacts youth's mental health
Legal status	Undocumented children and/or parents often live in fear of deportation; confront greater barriers to access health, financial, and health services; and are more likely to live in poverty
Family separation	The nature of the separation may determine its impact. Factors to consider are length of separation(s), whether children were separated from one or both parents, contact during separation, and quality and supportiveness of nonparent caretakers
Cultural/language brokering	Refers to the various activities that children do for their immigrant parents to facilitate adaptation to the new culture (i.e., translating documents, making health appointments, communicating with school officials, etc.)
Protective factor	
Parental socialization to culture of origin	Parents who engage in cultural/ethnic/racial socialization promote a sense of cultural/ethnic pride which, in turn, strengthens children's resilience
Family cohesion	Quality of family relationships, more so than family structure, is associated with positive youth outcomes (e.g., social skills, self-efficacy, self-esteem, etc.)
Family support	Social support from family, friends, neighborhoods, and communities play important roles in immigrant children's and parents' mental health

influence family dynamics and mental health [26]. Overall, acculturative stress has consistently been linked to decline in mental health among immigrant youth [27, 28] and adults [29, 30].

Discrimination

Immigrant parents and their children often also confront experiences of discrimination based on their immigration status and/or racial/ethnic background [31, 32]. One striking change faced by immigrants is the shift from being part of a cultural majority to a minority. These experiences may pose new challenges to the adaptation of immigrant families. For example, immigrant children recognize instances where they are discriminated by other peers and by adults [32, 33]. In addition, immigrant parents may experience discrimination looking for jobs or accessing services [34, 35]. There is evidence to suggest that the impact of these discriminatory experiences on the mental health of immigrant families is linked to the individual's interpretation of these events, suggesting that some may accept discrimination as part of the immigrant experience [31, 36]. Relatedly, a recent study of newcomer immigrant adolescents demonstrates that perceiving discrimination is linked to greater internalizing symptoms, depending on adolescents' appraisals. Those who appraised the discrimination event as more severe showed greater internalizing symptoms [37]. Intergenerational studies of discrimination further show that parents who perceive higher levels of discrimination have children who perceive higher levels [38]. Parents who perceive more discrimination may be driven to more actively engage in socialization practices that prepare their children to be aware of and cope with discrimination [39] and may be more likely to foster mistrust when parents perceive that they and their children were discriminated against [40]. Parental racial and cultural socialization can also play a protective role in the context of discrimination, providing children with knowledge about their heritage and racial history that serves to foster their self-esteem [41]. Taken together, evidence suggests that the impact of discrimination on the mental health of immigrant children and parents' roles are very significant and necessitate special attention in treatments and interventions [33, 36, 42, 43].

Violence Exposure

Exposure to trauma and violence before, during, and post-immigration is an important clinical consideration for immigrant families [5]. It is notable that communities and neighborhoods where immigrant families resettle may in fact expose them to new forms of violence [7, 44]. Studies suggest that general exposure to these experiences takes a toll on the mental health of immigrants, resulting most often in depression and post-traumatic stress disorder [44–47]. Emerging research in this area indicates that exposure to violence has a particularly pervasive negative impact on the psychopathology of immigrant youth, over and above experiencing acculturative stress [7].

Notably, although noted earlier that immigrant children may have some protections [20, 21], parent mental health can play a critical role in predicting child psychosocial adjustment in general [48] and specifically among refugee and war-affected immigrants [49]. A review of 100 studies found that parental post-traumatic stress symptoms are significantly related to child psychobiological vulnerability, including behavioral outcomes, internalizing symptoms, and hypothalamic-pituitary-adrenal functioning [50]. More research is necessary to examine whether the timing of exposure to trauma and violence relative to immigration uniquely affects mental health.

Legal Status

Legal conditions of entry into the new country also have important implications to the mental health and well-being of immigrant families. Specifically, immigrant families who are undocumented face additional barriers to living in, and navigating, the host country. Undocumented children and parents frequently live in fear of deportation; have a difficult time accessing educational, financial, and health services; and are more likely to live in poverty [51, 52]. These significant challenges have a detrimental effect on stress and psychopathology of immigrant children and parents [29, 53]. Continued attention to these issues is needed to fully understand the unique challenges of these families and the implications of changing laws and policies.

Transnational Families: Separation and Reunification

For many immigrant families, the migration process is marked by temporary and sometimes long-term separation from family members [54, 55]. A common challenge played out over months, years, and even decades is for immigrant families to endure the separation and, subsequently, adjust to reunification. Separations can occur in various forms. In sequential migration, one parent migrates first, followed by the other parent and children [56, 57]. In another pattern both parents migrate to find work, leaving their children behind in the care of family members such as grandparents, aunts, or uncles. "Astronaut families" are those where one parent accompanies the child (usually the mother) while the other parent stays behind, and "parachute kids" refer to those who are sent to stay with relatives or friends of the family in the new country to attend high school while both parents stay behind [58, 59]. Some patterns relate to the age of the children. For example, among families who can sustain the financial burden and have hopes for remittance, older children are sometimes sent abroad to work or study. At younger ages, some immigrant families engage in reverse migration whereby children born to mothers in the USA are sent back to the homeland to be raised by relatives until they are old enough to go to school [60]. Finally, immigrant families face separation when undocumented parents are sent back to the homeland while children remain [29]. In all of these patterns, there is potential for the separation and reunification process to undermine family relationships and challenge the adjustment of family members [55, 57, 61].

Separation is painful and difficult for both parents and children. Compared to immigrant children who have not experienced separation, children who have experienced separation report higher anxiety and depressive symptoms [55, 62]. Children may feel abandoned and lose trust in the parent, ultimately damaging the parent-child relationship [63]. Longer separations lead to greater risk for children to feel less connected to and identify less with their parents, and ultimately, to experience diminished family cohesion [55, 57].

Importantly, long-term effects of separation are not clear. One longitudinal study found that after 5 years, anxiety and depression lessened so that there was no longer a difference between children who experienced separation versus those who did not [55]. A study of young adults, reflecting on their experiences of separation during the migration process as children, found that some deeply appreciate the sacrifices their parents made to create a better life for them. They were grateful for their parents' hard work and acknowledged the upheavals their parents had to go through in order to establish themselves in a new country and pave the way for their children [57]. Some of these grown children, however, did not recover from the separation. For these children, feelings of estrangement from their parents persisted. Research suggests that the effects of separation, at least in the short term, and for a minority in the long-term, are not positive.

After separation, families look forward to reunification. Reunification, however, is marked by conflicting emotions. Children and parents report mixed emotions, ranging from happiness to hurt, and often complicated by jealousy toward new siblings or ambivalence and distance in the parent-child relationship [62]. Children have had to deal with the initial loss of a parent and then the subsequent loss of the caretaker who they may have grown quite attached to while their parent was away. During reunification children may experience a sense of disconnected from the parent and feel like the parent is a stranger [61, 64]. Parents may have difficulty, especially with a long separation, gaining the trust of their children and reestablishing authority [64]. If parents are experiencing difficulties and stressors in post-migration adaptation and adjustment, the added responsibilities and pressures of parenting can be another challenge. While parents may view their separation as a necessary sacrifice for the betterment of the family, their children may not immediately appreciate or agree with their parents' decision [61, 65]. Another challenge during reunification is reintegrating into a family with new family members [61]. There may be new stepparents and stepsiblings. New immigrant youth may be resentful of the time that parents had with the new partner and siblings who may have been born while the child was left behind [55]. Children who experience less positive and more disruptive reunions may act out [66] and do more poorly in school [67, 68].

In sum, the emotional, psychological, and relational consequences associated with separation and reunion during the migration process depend on various factors: developmental period during which the separation occurred (e.g., infancy, toddlerhood, childhood, or adolescence), length of separation, whether children were separated from one or both parents, how much contact was maintained, reasons for migration, extent of acculturative stress experienced, and quality and supportiveness of the relationship with nonparent caretakers. At least in the short term, separation and reunification are stressful disruptions for immigrant family relationships. Over time, although there is a wide range of variability in context and experience, most families do ultimately restabilize and are able to function [66]. Future research should focus on potential long-term effects and factors that predict more positive reunification experiences and subsequent adjustment.

Case Study

Elisa is a mother of two from El Salvador. Her husband migrated to the USA first, and his distance and lack of communication were ultimately connected to him having built a new relationship and family in the USA and, in essence, abandoning his family in El Salvador. Elisa subsequently migrated alone to improve the life of her children, ages 8 (Vanessa) and 11 (Mauricio), whom she left behind, to protect them from the uncertainty and difficulty of crossing the border into the USA. She sought out domestic work, and the act of sending remittances made the distress and pain of the separation from her children more bearable. However, her ability to find work has been unstable, so she is sometimes struggling to make ends meet and send her earnings back home. She is finally able to bring her son, Mauricio, to the USA after 1 year. He travels across the border with his uncle. Instead of bringing relief, Elisa feels more worried and overwhelmed because after such a long separation, Mauricio is angry and defiant, and she is unable to supervise him when she is working. She worries that he will get involved with local gang activity. Meanwhile, Elisa's absence in El Salvador is being felt more acutely by her remaining child, Vanessa, who continues to live with her ailing grandmother andhasbecome increasingly anxious and clingy, not wanting to be by herself at any time.

Cultural and Language Brokering

Cultural and language brokering refers to the activities that children do for their immigrant parents to facilitate adaption to the new culture. Children may translate documents; facilitate communication with doctors, businesses, and government agencies; file taxes; make medical- and health-related appointments; answer the telephone; and communicate with school officials [69, 70]. Children act as translators and advocates in helping their parents navigate through legal, medical, financial, and interpersonal issues and interactions [69], and this can include the therapeutic context.

One of the major questions related to the experience of cultural brokering is whether it is related to more positive or negative child development and family relations. On the one hand, cultural brokering could lead to parentification or role reversal—taking on adult responsibilities that may be premature and developmentally inappropriate [71, 72]. Because of the linguistic and cognitive demands required, younger children may experience brokering as more stressful than older adolescents [73]. Another important clinical consideration for some immigrant families is the type and frequency of obligations placed on children which extend into areas that are complicated and consequential [69]. On the other hand, scholars have suggested that cultural brokering provides a sense of responsibility, where youth have the opportunity to view themselves as making valuable contribution to the family. In this view, cultural brokering is a normative aspect of the immigrant children's experience that does not lead to dysfunction [74, 75].

Thus far, empirical findings support both views. Some studies find that adolescents of immigrant families who engage in more cultural brokering also report greater family conflict and family stress [76–78], less self-esteem and self-efficacy [79], and greater internalizing and externalizing problems [69, 80]. Others find that adolescents perceive cultural brokering as a "primarily positive experience" [75, 81] and is related to greater perceived competence [82], stronger ethnic identity [83], and greater empathy and transcultural perspective-taking [84]. Attention to age of the child (e.g., is cultural brokering happening as a young child or during adolescence), brokering domain, and interactions with other factors such as parent support will be important for future research to clarify the impact of cultural brokering on psychosocial development for immigrant youth.

Case Study

The Chu family immigrated from Vietnam 5 years ago with their first two children, and their third child was born in the USA. The family's oldest daughter, Mai, is 12 years old and often plays the role of caretaker to her younger siblings and language broker for her parents. As a language broker, she frequently completes school forms and translates school letters for her parents. Most recently, her grades started falling and she appears to be sullen and withdrawn. These changes were precipitated by her mother's cancer diagnosis, for which Mai has had to attend multiple doctor's appointments. During these appointments she often participates by translating and interacting with medical staff to understand and explain her mother's physical health issues to the doctors and to her mother. Meanwhile, she tries to cope with her mother's diagnosis. Mai explains that she feels proud to be in a position to help her mother during this difficult time.

Acculturation Gaps

One of the most studied areas of immigrant families is the focus on parent-child differences in acculturation. Since children from immigrant families tend to acquire the values and behaviors of the new culture at a faster rate than their parents, a large difference in values and behaviors may result [85]. This parent-child acculturation difference has been termed *the acculturation gap* [85], *acculturation dissonance* [86], and *acculturative family distancing* [87]. These scholars have proposed that greater acculturation gaps are detrimental to child development by changing the family dynamics in several ways. Parents' may lose their ability to guide their children in important areas of life, such as academics [4, 86]. Parents and children may develop dual frames of reference and, subsequently, feelings of alienation from one another [88], which may lead to greater family conflict [89].

Research on acculturation in general and on specific components (e.g., family obligation, autonomy expectation, and parental warmth and control) shows that the parent-child acculturation gap is related to parent-child conflict and child maladjustment (e.g., greater internalizing and externalizing symptoms, lower life satisfaction, and lower self-esteem) [89–91]. One study found that a gap in the heritage culture dimension was related to poorer adolescent adjustment, but a gap in the mainstream culture dimension was not [92]. A review of the acculturation gap literature suggests that the relation between acculturation gaps and adolescent adjustment is more complex than is usually presented, and the relations are not always consistent [93, 94]. Importantly, Telzer's [94] review suggests that the acculturation process and resulting acculturation gaps do not inevitably occur, and when they do occur, they do not necessarily lead to greater family conflict or child maladjustment. These findings are important for expanding our view of immigrant families beyond their roles in contexts defined solely by acculturation gaps and conflicts.

Even with the acculturation gap developing over time, immigrant parents remain a primary source of support for their children. Specifically, parents are often the channel through which an immigrant child can connect with society, maneuver a new culture, and remain connected to family cultural heritage [97]. Cultural and racial socializing practices can foster connection with cultural heritage (i.e., identity, belongingness, pride), reinforce their resilience when faced with discrimination and contribute to better adjustment in terms of self-esteem, mental health (e.g., depression) and school performance for immigrant youth [40, 95, 96, 98, 99, 100, 101].

Case Study

Abdi is a 15-year-old male whose parents immigrated from Somalia when he was a baby. Now, as a teenager, while his parents dress in traditional clothing, his manner and dress are more aligned with his American classmates in high school. His parents express frustration with his disobedience and concern that he is spending time with peers who are getting into trouble after school. Moreover, Abdi is failing most of his classes. Abdi's father works the graveyard shift as a security guard, and his mother feels isolated because she has little support and has had difficulty finding employment. She often cries, thinking about leaving her homeland and how far away she is from her extended family. Abdi feels that his parents do not understand him. He knows very little about his parents' immigration experience and the treacherous journey they faced escaping civil war.

Family Conflict

Two types of family conflict have been studied in immigrant families: minor, everyday conflict, and more serious, acculturation-based conflict. Everyday conflict, or "minor" arguments over issues such as household chores and schoolwork, has been studied primarily among European American families. The few studies including immigrant families of Mexican, Chinese, and Filipino heritage show that these adolescents engaged in similar types of everyday conflicts as their European American counterparts, such as household chores and schoolwork, at low to moderate levels [102–104]. Conflict over everyday issues is viewed as normative, temporary, and functional, as it realigns the parent-adolescent relationship [105] and facilitates the development of autonomy (or individuation) for youth of various cultural backgrounds [103, 106–108]. Further, it is argued that this realignment ultimately establishes a parent-adolescent relationship that is "less contentious, more egalitarian, and less volatile" [107, p. 88].

In addition to everyday conflict, acculturation-based conflict, or more "serious" arguments that are rooted in cultural value differences (i.e., acculturation gaps) between parents and children, has been studied primarily among Asian- and Latino-heritage families (both characterized as emphasizing family interdependence) and is viewed as a threat to relatedness with parents rather than the normative assertion of autonomy [71]. As noted earlier, acculturation gaps do not necessarily erupt into conflict [94]. But when they do, this conflict is associated with negative adjustment for adolescents [89–91]. Thus, in contrast to everyday conflict, acculturation-based conflict tends to be viewed more negatively and is rarely considered to be developmentally normative or adaptive [71, 85, 86]. Importantly, acculturation-based conflict has been found to be a better predictor of adjustment compared to everyday conflict for Chinese-heritage immigrant adolescents [109].

There is some evidence, however, that acculturation-based conflict in adolescence, similar to everyday conflict, may not have negative long-term consequences—at least for some families. For instance, one study found that acculturation-related conflicts were common among Korean American college students, particularly around challenges with communication, given a lack of fluency in a shared language, between parents and adolescents, as well as conflicts based around academic demands prioritized over all else [110]. However, Kang and colleagues [110] conclude that although relationships between parents and adolescents were often difficult, by emerging adulthood a majority of Korean Americans could reconcile their difficult relationships and come to a greater understanding and appreciation of their parents. They were able to consider their parents' perspective, empathize, and reinterpret conflicts with parents in a constructive way. They could see, for instance, the great sacrifice their parents endured so their children could have a better life. Future studies should examine how immigrant youth make meaning of family conflict as they get older and focus on implications for their current relationships with their parents and their long-term adjustment.

Case Study

The Mazdani family immigrated from Iran. The father is a doctor and the mother was a nurse in Iran but, since coming to the USA, has taken a position as an interpreter at the local hospital. Their daughter Anahita is enrolled in all Advanced Placement classes at her high school and is already planning for medical school. Over time, her anxiety has increased, and like her mother, she has started to have panic attacks and, subsequently, began limiting her after-school and social activities. Anahita and her mother spend almost all of their time together and are in constant everyday conflict about chores, schoolwork, and going out with friends, which her mother restricts. Anahita's mother regularly uses shame and the pressure to uphold family honor, to influence her daughter's choices. Mrs. Mazdani often tells Anahita how she lost everything she worked for when the family moved to the USA. Anahita feels the pressure to become a doctor, to honor her mother and father's sacrifices on her behalf. Anahita feels that despite her academic achievements, her grades are insufficient; she feels overwhelmed and constantly preoccupied with the stress of college applications and overwhelmed that she will let her family down if she is unable to achieve a level that is satisfactory to them.

Prevention and Intervention for Immigrant Families

There are a number of major challenges related to prevention and intervention for immigrant families. There are numerous potential barriers to service access, including acculturative, cultural, and linguistic barriers, and meeting everyone's, sometimes quite varying, needs. Acculturative gaps between parents and children may play a significant role. For example, therapy provided in the language of origin may be appropriate for parents but not for children who are not necessarily fluent in that language. Values and adherence to cultural norms may also be quite different for parents and children.

Bicultural Effectiveness Training (BET), a family intervention for Latino families, addresses the acculturative gap, blending structural family systems therapy with cultural considerations for families that reside in a multicultural context [111]. The BET intervention frames family conflict as a cultural conflict, offers a transcultural perspective, and encourages cross alliances by accepting biculturalism among different generations and cultures within the family context [112].

The Strengthening of Intergenerational/Intercultural Ties in Immigrant Families (SITIF) is geared toward immigrant parents of school-aged children [113]. This community-based intervention aims to promote greater awareness of potential intergenerational cultural misunderstandings and conflicts, increase parents' empathy for their children's cultural experiences, and teach parents specific parenting skills such as strategies for more effective parent-child communication. An initial pilot study with Chinese immigrant parents showed that at the 3-month follow-up, this intervention led to a greater sense of parental control and more positive relationship with their children [114].

Falicov [115] suggests the importance of using four domains—migration, ecological context, family organization, and the family life cycle (MECA)—as a helpful tool for practitioners to understand the processes relevant to immigrant families. Attention to these domains can be important across socioecological levels, whereby schools and communities could also be targeted in family intervention efforts, in order to improve accessibility, engagement, and overall effectiveness in supporting immigrant families [116].

Case Study

The Wong family immigrated from southern China. Since coming to the USA, Mr. and Mrs. Wong attained jobs working in a restaurant. Their son Henry is enrolled in 5th grade and is having difficulty in school because of language barriers and challenges with making friends. In the past 6 months, Henry has had increased sadness and lost interest in his favorite hobbies and school. However, Henry does not tell his parents about his struggle. Instead he acts out and withdraws from all family communication. Mrs. Wong sees that her son is struggling with school and communication so she decides to follow her friend's advice to enroll in the 8-week Strengthening of Intergenerational/ Intercultural Ties in Immigrant Families (SITIF) parenting class, taking her husband along with her.

During the first few sessions, the focus of the program was to develop awareness about themselves, their emotions, and about cross-cultural differences that may be uniquely experienced by each family member. The next several sessions were devoted to behavioral parenting skills training. Mr. and Mrs. Wong learned skills on how to be empathic toward Henry, with the goal of helping him to communicate better. They learned about creating structure, rules, limits, and a reward system for Henry. The session that followed focused on coping with stress, including the immigration-related stressors that the Wongs had endured. The final class was devoted to reviewing and integrating the material learned during the 8-week course. Mr. and Mrs. Wong reviewed what they had learned and reflected on how to apply their new skills in supporting Henry with his communication and school difficulties.

Family Strengths and Protective Factors

Current research on family strengths and protective factors offers a useful vantage point for detailing factors that support positive outcomes for immigrant families and their youth. The notion of resilience focuses on an individual's ability to adapt in the context of adversity [117]. The study of resilience has expanded to include family, interpersonal, and sociocultural factors through frameworks such as the resiliency model [118] and a family resilience perspective [117, 119]. These perspectives offer valuable considerations for treatment of immigrant families. Specifically, the shift to viewing families as facing immigration-related stressors can frame struggles as a product of contextual factors rather than a result of a dysfunctional family. Moreover, strengths, resources, and protective factors can be incorporated into the conceptualization of a family's functioning, taking into consideration the ways in which the immigrant family system interacts with other ecological contexts they encounter [120]. Family belief systems, organizational patterns, and communication/problem-solving can play an important role in family resilience [117]. Meaning making can be an especially important task to help connect family members in facing challenges and adversities together and developing a family process of resilience [121].

It is important to consider the effects of both family structure and the quality of family relationships on child outcomes among immigrant populations. For example, in a large longitudinal study of immigrant youth ($n=2063$), family structure was found to be predictive of youth outcomes (e.g., educational performance, self-esteem, and depression), whereas the quality of family relationships (e.g., family cohesion and parent-child conflict) was found to be even stronger predictors of self-esteem and depression compared to family structure as a predictor [122]. Family cohesion serves as a protective factor for depression [123] and has been found to be associated with improvements in children's social skills (e.g., problem-solving and self-efficacy) [124]. Leidy and colleagues [124] suggest that "efforts to enhance positive parenting and effective family functioning must consider how best to help parents navigate acculturation gaps" (p. 11). They found that there are multiple factors that impact immigrant parents' ability to parent and foster family cohesion (e.g., acculturative differences, challenges to get involved in child's education, reduced access to extended family, and discrimination). When intervening with immigrant families, it is pertinent to explore how to empower parents to overcome these challenges that may impede their ability to facilitate protective family processes that will in turn promote family resilience.

Various family strengths have been identified for specific immigrant populations that should also be taken into consideration when intervening with clinical problems. Xia et al. [125] identified family strengths among new Chinese immigrants to include family support, social support, communication, and spiritual well-being. Among Japanese immigrant mothers and their adult daughters, family strengths of actively pursuing strategies to improve language acculturation challenges (i.e., receiving help, asking for clarification from parent, using humor, and aiding in improving mother's language) were found [126]. These simple yet innovative strategies could be beneficial in promoting enhanced communication among immigrant families who may be acculturating at different rates.

Another major source of strength for immigrant families is derived from social support. Ayón and Bou Ghosn Naddy [127] described family, friends, neighbors, and the community as the most substantial categories that emerged for sources of social support for Latino immigrant families in their focus groups. Interestingly, it is evident that immigrant families may seek strength and support from various levels of their ecology as suggested in Bronfenbrenner's ecological model. Research suggests that social support has a protective effect on long-term immigrants' mental health outcomes [128]. In a large sample of Asian immigrants ($n = 1639$), the benefits of social support from relatives and friends were delineated such that social support partially mediated the relationship between acculturative stress and depressive symptoms; in other words, those who reported lower levels of acculturative stress reported higher social support and, in turn, experienced fewer depressive symptoms [30].

Taking into consideration the strong evidence of the protective effects of social support on immigrant outcomes, it is advisable to encourage opportunities for families to expand their networks of support to include various levels within the family context, schools, neighborhood, and larger community. However, practitioners who aim to encourage immigrant clients to build their social support network should understand the various barriers that may impede this process. In a study of Latina immigrants who reported changes in social isolation after moving to the USA, the following barriers to establishing social networks were identified: socioeconomic challenges (i.e., demanding jobs and relationship envy about employment), environmental barriers (i.e., space and transportation deficits), and psychosocial barriers (i.e., trust concerns and emotional strains [129]. Immigrant families may benefit from assistance in navigating these barriers to accessing social support networks. Researchers suggest incorporating opportunities for the construction of informal social supports where immigrant families can learn from one another [130].

Conclusion

Immigrant families confront unique hurdles before, during, and long after immigration. These challenges have a significant impact on the children and parents' mental health and well-being and consequently should be considered and integrated into the conceptualization and delivery of mental health interventions for this population. Understanding immigrant family strengths and resilience processes is crucial to inform interventions that help immigrants learn how to capitalize on factors that contribute to positive outcomes and adaptive coping to immigration stressors. Practitioners can benefit from applying a multisystem approach for interventions that considers the complexity of family strengths, functioning, and resilience in the face of adversity.

References

1. Camarota SA, Zeigler K. One in five U.S. residents speaks foreign language at home, record 61.8 million: Spanish, Chinese, and Arabic speakers grew most since 2010; 2014. Retrieved at: http://cis.org/record-one-in-five-us-residents-speaks-language-other-than-english-at-home.
2. Mather M. Children in immigrant families chart new path. Washington, DC: Population Reference Bureau; 2009. Retrieved from http://www.prb.org/pdf09/immigrantchildren.pdf.
3. Pumariega AJ, Rothe E. Leaving no children or families outside: the challenges of immigration. Am J Orthopsychiatry. 2010;80(4):505–15. doi:10.1111/j.1939-0025.2010.01053.x.

4. Suárez-Orozco C, Suárez-Orozco MM. Children of immigrants. Cambridge, MA: Harvard University Press; 2001.
5. Rettger JP, Kletter H, Carrion V. Trauma and acculturative stress. In: Patel SG, Reicherter D, editors. Psychotherapy for immigrant youth. New York, NY: Springer Science + Business Media; 2015.
6. Staudenmeyer A, Macciomei E, del Cid M, Patel SG. Immigrant youth life stressors. In: Patel SG, Reicherter D, editors. Psychotherapy for immigrant youth. New York, NY: Springer Science + Business Media; 2015.
7. Gudiño OG, Nadeem E, Kataoka SH, Lau AS. Relative impact of violence exposure and immigrant stressors on Latino youth psychopathology. J Commun Psychol. 2011;39(3):316–35. doi:10.1002/jcop.20435.
8. Bronfenbrenner U, Morris PA. The bioecological model of human development. In: Damon W, Lerner RM, editors. Handbook of child psychology, Theoretical models of human development, vol. 1. 6th ed. Hoboken, NJ: Wiley; 2006. p. 793–828.
9. Kia-Keating M, Dowdy E, Morgan ML, Noam GG. Protecting and promoting: an integrative conceptual model for healthy development of adolescents. J Adolesc Health. 2011;48(3):220–8. doi:10.1016/j.jadohealth.2010.08.006.
10. Kuperminc GP, Wilkins NJ, Roche C, Alvarez-Jimenez A. Risk, resilience, and positive development. In: Villarruel FA, Carlo G, Grau JM, Azmitia M, Cabrera N, Chahin TJ, editors. Handbook of US Latino psychology: developmental and community based perspectives. Thousand Oaks, CA: Sage; 2009. p. 213–34.
11. Bronfenbrenner U. The ecology of human development: experiments by nature and design. Cambridge, MA: Harvard University Press; 1979.
12. Masten AS. Ordinary magic: resilience processes in development. Am Psychol. 2001;56(3):227–38. doi:10.1177/0272431608324477.
13. Rutter M. Psychosocial resilience and protective mechanisms. Am J Orthopsychiatry. 1987;57(3):316–31. doi:10.1111/j.1939-0025.1987.tb03541.x.
14. Sandler I. Quality and ecology of adversity as common mechanisms of risk and resilience. Am J Community Psychol. 2001;29(1):19–61. doi:10.1023/A:1005237110505.
15. Ford DL, Lerner R. Developmental systems theory: an integrative approach. Newbury Park, CA: Sage; 1992.
16. Weine SM. Family roles in refugee youth resettlement from a prevention perspective. Child Adolesc Psychiatr Clin N Am. 2009;17:515–32. doi:10.1016/j.chc.2008.02.006.
17. American Psychological Association (APA). Guidelines on multicultural education, training, research, practice, and organizational change for psychologists; 2002. Retrieved from: http://www.apa.org/pi/oema/resources/policy/multicultural-guideline.pdf
18. Alegria M, Canino G, Stinson FS, Grant BF. Nativity and DSM-IV psychiatric disorders among Puerto Ricans, Cuban Americans, and non-Latino whites in the United States: results from the national epidemiologic survey on alcohol and related conditions. J Clin Psychiatry. 2006;67(1):56–65. http://dx.doi.org/10.4088/JCP.v67n0109.
19. Coll C, Marks AK, editors. The immigrant paradox in children and adolescents: Is becoming American a developmental risk? Washington, DC: American Psychological Association; 2012.
20. Bennet AC, Brewer KC, Rankin KM. The association of child mental health conditions and parent mental health status among U.S. children, 2007. Matern Child Health J. 2012;16:1266–75. doi:10.1007/s10995-011-0888-4.
21. Degboe A, Belue R, Hillemeire M. Parental immigrant status and adolescent mental health in the United States: Do racial/ethnic differences exist? Child Adolesc Mental Health. 2012;17(4):209–15. doi:10.1111/j.1475-3588.2011.00636.x.
22. Martinez CR, McClure HH, Eddy JM, Wilson DM. Time in the U.S. residency and the social, behavioral, and emotional adjustment of Latino immigrant families. Hisp J Behav Sci. 2011;33(3):323–49. doi:10.1177/0739986311411281.
23. Williams CL, Berry JW. Primary prevention of acculturative stress among refugees: Application of psychological theory and practice. Am Psychol. 1991;46(6):632–41. http://dx.doi.org/10.1037/0003-066X.46.6.632.

24. Castillo LG, Cano M, Chen SW, Blucker RT, Olds TS. Family conflict and intragroup marginalization as predictors of acculturative stress in Latino college students. Int J Stress Manag. 2008;15(1):43–52. doi:10.1037/1072-5245.15.1.43.
25. Sciarra DT, Ponterotto JG. Counseling the Hispanic bilingual family: challenges to the therapeutic process. Psychotherapy: Theory, Research, Practice, Training. 1991;28(3):473–79.
26. Miranda AO, Bilot JM, Peluso PR, Berman K, Van Meek LG. Latino families: the relevance of the connection among acculturation, family dynamics, and health for family counseling research and practice. Family J. 2006;14(3):268–74.
27. Katsiaficas D, Suárez-Orozco C, Sirin SR, Gupta T. Mediators of the relationship between acculturative stress and internalization symptoms for immigrant origin youth. Cult Divers Ethn Minor Psychol. 2013;9(1):27–37. doi:10.1037/a0031094.
28. Sirin SR, Gupta T, Ryce P, Katsiaficas D, Suárez-Orozco C, Rogers-Sirin L. Understanding the role of social support in trajectories of mental health symptoms for immigrant adolescents. J Appl Dev Psychol. 2013;34:199–207. doi:10.1016/j.appdev.2013.04.004.
29. Arbona C, Olvera N, Rodriguez N, Hagan J, Linares A, Wiesner M. Acculturative stress among documented and undocumented Latino immigrants in the United States. Hisp J Behav Sci. 2010;32(3):362–84. doi:10.1177/0739986310373210.
30. Xu L, Chi I. Acculturative stress and depressive symptoms among Asian immigrants in the United States: the roles of social support and negative interaction. Asian Am J Psychol. 2013;4(3):217–26. doi:10.1037/s0030167.
31. Edwards LM, Romero AJ. Coping with discrimination among Mexican descent adolescents. Hisp J Behav Sci. 2008;30:24–39. doi:10.1177/0739986307311431.
32. Zhou M, Xiong YS. The multifaceted American experiences of the children of Asian immigrants: lessons for segmented assimilation. Ethn Racial Stud Special Issue: The Second Generation in Early Adulthood. 2005;28:1119–52. doi:10.1080/01419870500224455.
33. Huynh V, Fuligni AJ. Discrimination hurts: the academic, psychological, and physical well-being of adolescents. J Res Adolesc. 2010;20(4):916–41. doi:10.1111/j.1532-7795.2010.00670.x.
34. Araujo Dawson B. Discrimination, stress, and acculturation among Dominican immigrant women. Hisp J Behav Sci. 2009;31(1):96–111. http://dx.doi.org/10.1177/0739986308327502.
35. Tran AGTT, Lee RM, Burgess DJ. Perceived discrimination and substance use in Hispanic/Latino, African-born Black, and Southeast Asian immigrants. Cult Divers Ethn Minor Psychol. 2010;16(2):226–36. http://dx.doi.org/10.1037/a0016344.
36. Ayón C, Marsiglia F, Bermudez-Parsai M. Latino family mental health: exploring the role of discrimination and familismo. J Commun Psychol. 2010;38(6):742–56. doi:10.1002/jcop.20392.
37. Patel SG, Tabb KM, Strambler MJ, Eltareb F. Newcomer immigrant adolescents and ambiguous discrimination: the role of cognitive appraisal. J Adolesc Res. 2015;30(1):7–30. doi:10.1177/0743558414546717.
38. Juang LP, Alvarez AN. Family, school, and neighborhood: links to Chinese American adolescent perceptions of racial/ethnic discrimination. Asian Am J Psychol. 2011;2(1):1–12. doi:10.1037/a0023107.
39. Stevenson Jr HC, Cameron R, Herrero-Taylor T, Davis GY. Development of the teenager experience of racial socialization scale: correlates of race-related socialization frequency from the perspective of Black youth. J Black Psychol. 2002;28(2):84–106. doi:10.1177/0095798402028002002.
40. Hughes D, Johnson DJ. Correlates in children's experiences of parents' racial socialization behaviors. J Marriage Fam. 2001;63:981–95.
41. Hughes D, Smith EP, Stevenson HC, Rodriguez J, Johnson DJ, Spicer P. Parents' ethnic-racial socialization practices: a review of research and directions for future study. Dev Psychol. 2006;42(5):747–70. doi:10.1037/0012-1649.42.5.747.
42. Llácer A, Del Amo J, García-Fulgueiras A, Ibáñez-Rojo V, García-Pino R, Jarrín I, et al. Discrimination and mental health in Ecuadorian immigrants in Spain. J Epidemiol Commun Health. 2009;63(9):766–72. http://dx.doi.org/10.1136/jech.2008.085530.

43. Noh S, Kaspar V, Wickrama KAS. Overt and subtle racial discrimination and mental health: preliminary findings for Korean immigrants. Am J Public Health. 2007;97(7):1269–74. http://dx.doi.org/10.2105/AJPH.2005.085316.
44. Jaycox L, Stein B, Kataoka SH, Wong M, Fink A, Escudero P, Zaragoza C. Violence exposure, posttraumatic stress disorder and depressive symptoms among recent immigrant schoolchildren. Am Acad Child Adolesc Psychiatry. 2012;41(9):1104–10. doi:10.1097/00004583-200209000-00011.
45. Bridges AJ, de Arellano MA, Rheingold AA, Danielson CK, Silcott L. Trauma exposure, mental health, and service utilization rates among immigrant and United States-born Hispanic youth: results from the Hispanic family study. Psychol Trauma. 2010;2(1):40–8. http://dx.doi.org/10.1037/a0019021.
46. Fortuna LR, Porche MV, Alegria M. Political violence, psychosocial trauma, and the context of mental health services use among immigrant Latinos in the United States. Ethnic Health. 2008;13(5):435–63. http://dx.doi.org/10.1080/13557850701837286.
47. Rousseau C, Drapeau A. Premigration exposure to political violence among independent immigrants and its association with emotional distress. J Nerv Ment Dis. 2004;192(12):852–6. doi:10.1097/01.nmd.0000146740.66351.23.
48. Beardslee WR, Gladstone TR, O'Connor EE. Transmission and prevention of mood disorders among children of affectively ill parents: a review. J Am Acad Child Adolesc Psychiatry. 2011;50:1098–109.
49. Porterfield K, Akinsulure-Smith A, Benson M, Betancourt T, Ellis H, Kia-Keating M, Miller K. Resilience and recovery after war: refugee children and families in the United States. Report of the APA task force on the psychosocial effects of war on children and families who are refugees from armed conflict residing in the United States. Washington, DC: American Psychological Association; 2010.
50. Leen-Feldner EW, Feldner MT, Knapp A, Bunaciu L, Blumenthal H, Amstadter AB. Offspring psychological and biological correlates of parental posttraumatic stress: review of the literature and research agenda. Clin Psychol Rev. 2013;33:1106–33. doi:10.1016/j.cpr.2013.09.001.
51. Gonzales R, Suárez-Orozco C, Dedios-Sanguineti MC. No place to belong: conceptualizing concepts of mental health among undocumented immigrant youth in the United States. Am Behav Sci. 2013;57(8):1174–99.
52. Suárez-Orozco C, Yoshikawa H, Teranishi R, Suárez-Orozco MM. Growing up in the shadows: the developmental implications of unauthorized status. Harv Educ Rev. 2011;81(3):438–72.
53. Suárez-Orozco C, Yoshikawa H. Undocumented status: implications for child development, policy, and ethical research. In: Hernández MG, Nguyen J, Saetermoe CL, Suárez-Orozco C, editors. Frameworks and ethics for research with immigrants. New Directions for child and adolescent development, vol. 141. Ann Arbor, MI: Wiley Periodicals; 2013. p. 61–78.
54. Hernandez DJ, Denton NA, Macartney SE. Family circumstances of children in immigrant families: looking to the future of America. In: Lansford JE, Deater-Deckard K, Bornstein MH, editors. Immigrant families in contemporary society. New York, NY: Guilford; 2007. p. 9–29.
55. Suárez-Orozco C, Bang HJ, Kim HY. I felt like my heart was staying behind: psychological implications of family separations and reunifications for immigrant youth. J Adolesc Res. 2011;26(2):222–57. doi:10.1177/0743558410376830.
56. Rusch D, Reyes K. Examining the effects of Mexican serial migration and family separations on acculturative stress, depression, and family functioning. Hisp J Behav Sci. 2013;35(2):139–58. doi:10.1177/0739986312467292.
57. Smith A, Lalonde RN, Johnson S. Serial migration and its implications for the parent-child relationship: a retrospective analysis of the experiences of the children of Caribbean immigrants. Cult Divers Ethn Minor Psychol. 2004;10(2):107–22. http://dx.doi.org/10.1037/1099-9809.10.2.107.
58. Lee H-H, Friedlander ML. Predicting depressive symptoms from acculturative family distancing: a study of Taiwanese parachute kids in adulthood. Cult Divers Ethn Minor Psychol. 2014;20(3):458–62. http://dx.doi.org/10.1037/0022-0167.51.2.263.

59. Tsong Y, Liu Y. Parachute kids and astronaut families. In: Tewari N, Alvarez AN, editors. Asian American psychology: current perspectives. New York, NY: Routledge/Taylor & Francis Group; 2009. p. 365–79.
60. Kwong K, Chung H, Sun L, Chou JC, Taylor-Shih A. Factors associated with reverse-migration separation among a cohort of low-income Chinese immigrant families in New York City. Soc Work Health Care. 2009;48(3):348–59. doi:10.1080/00981380802599174.
61. Foner N, Dreby J. Relations between the generations in immigrant families. Annu Rev Sociol. 2011;37:545–64. doi:10.1146/annurev-soc-081309-150030.
62. Suárez-Orozco C, Todorova ILG, Louie J. Making up for lost time: the experience of separation and reunification among immigrant families. Fam Process. 2002;41(4):625–43. doi:10.1111/j.1545-5300.2002.00625.x.
63. Glasgow GF, Gouse-Sheese J. Theme of rejection and abandonment in group work with Caribbean adolescents. Soc Work Groups. 1995;17(4):3–27. doi:10.1300/J009v17n04_02.
64. Mitrani VB, Santisteban DA, Muir JA. Addressing immigration-related separations in Hispanic families with a behavior-problem adolescent. Am J Orthopsychiatry. 2004;74(3):219–29. http://dx.doi.org/10.1037/0002-9432.74.3.219.
65. Zhou M. Conflict, coping, and reconciliation: intergenerational relations in Chinese immigrant families. In: Foner N, editor. Across generations: immigrant families in America. New York, NY: New York University Press; 2009. p. 21–46.
66. Suárez-Orozco C, Suárez-Orozco MM. The psychosocial experience of immigration. In: LeVine RA, editor. Psychological anthropology: a reader on self in culture. Malden, MA: Wiley-Blackwell; 2010. p. 329–44.
67. Gindling TH, Poggio S. Family separation and the educational success of immigrant children. Policy Brief. Baltimore, MD: University of Maryland; 2009.
68. Suárez-Orozco C, Suárez-Orozco MM, Todorova I. Learning a new land: immigrant students in American society. Cambridge, MA: Belknap Press/Harvard University Press; 2008.
69. Chao RK. The prevalence and consequences of adolescents' language brokering for their immigrant parents. In: Bornstein MH, Cote LR, editors. Acculturation and parent-child relationships: measurement and development. Mahwah, NJ: Lawrence Erlbaum; 2006. p. 271–96.
70. Morales A, Hanson WE. Language brokering: an integrative review of the literature. Hisp J Behav Sci. 2005;27(4):471–503. doi:10.1177/0739986305281333.
71. Portes A, Rumbaut R. Legacies: the story of the immigrant second generation. Berkeley: University of California Press; 2001.
72. Titzmann PF. Growing up too soon? Parentification among immigrant and native adolescents in Germany. J Youth Adolesc. 2012;41(7):880–93. doi:10.1007/s10964-011-9711-1.
73. Weisskirch RS, Alva SA. Language brokering and the acculturation of Latino children. Hisp J Behav Sci. 2002;24:369–78.
74. Orellana MF. The work kids do: Mexican and Central American immigrant children's contributions to households and schools in California. Harv Educ Rev. 2001;71(3):366–90.
75. Orellana MF, Dorner L, Pulido L. Assessing assets: Immigrant youth's work as family translators or "para-phrasers". Soc Probl. 2003;50(4):505–24.
76. Hua JM, Costigan CL. The familial context of adolescent language brokering within immigrant Chinese families in Canada. J Youth Adolesc. 2012;41:894–906. http://dx.doi.org/10.1007/s10964-011-9682-2.
77. Jones C, Trickett EJ. Immigrant adolescents behaving as culture brokers: a study of families from the former Soviet Union. J Soc Psychol. 2005;145:405–27. doi:10.3200/SOCP.145.4.405-428.
78. Trickett EJ, Jones CJ. Adolescent culture brokering and family functioning: a study of families from Vietnam. Cult Divers Ethn Minor Psychol. 2007;13(2):143–50. doi:10.1037/1099-9809.13.2.143.
79. Oznobishin O, Kurman J. Parent–child role reversal and psychological adjustment among immigrant youth in Israel. J Fam Psychol. 2009;23(3):405–15. http://dx.doi.org/10.1037/a0015811.

80. Martinez CR, McClure H, Eddy J. Language brokering contexts and behavioral and emotional adjustment among Latino parents and adolescents. J Early Adolesc. 2008;36:124–43. doi:10.1177/0272431608324477.
81. McQuillan J, Tse L. Child language brokering in linguistic minority communities: effects on cultural interaction, cognition, and literacy. Lang Educ. 1995;9(3):195–215. doi:10.1080/09500789509541413.
82. Buriel R, Perez W, De Ment TL, Chavez DV, Moran VR. The relationship of language brokering to academic performance, biculturalism, and self-efficacy among Latino adolescents. Hisp J Behav Sci.1998;20(3):283–97. doi:10.1177/07399863980203001.
83. Weisskirch RS. The relationship of language brokering to ethnic identity for Latino early adolescents. Hisp J Behav Sci. 2005;27(3):286–99. doi:10.1177/0739986305277931.
84. Guan S-SA, Greenfield PM, Orellana MF. Translating into understanding: language brokering and prosocial development in emerging adults from immigrant families. J Adolesc Res. 2014;29(3):331–55. doi:10.1177/0743558413520223.
85. Kwak K. Adolescents and their parents: a review of intergenerational family relations for immigrant and non-immigrant families. Hum Dev. 2003;46(2–3):15–136. http://dx.doi.org/10.1159/000068581.
86. Portes A, Rumbaut RG. Immigrant America: a portrait. Berkeley, CA: Univeristy of California Press; 1996.
87. Hwang Y. Investigating the role of identity and gender in technology mediated learning. Behav Inform Technol. 2010;29(3):305–19. doi:10.1080/01449290902915754.
88. Qin DB. 'Our child doesn't talk to us anymore': alienation in immigrant Chinese families. Anthropol Educ Quart. 2006;37(2):162–79. doi:10.1525/aeq.2006.37.2.162.
89. Phinney JS, Ong A, Madden T. Cultural values and intergenerational value discrepancies in immigrant and non-immigrant families. Child Dev. 2000;71(2):528–39. doi:10.1111/1467-8624.00162.
90. Juang LP, Syed M, Takagi M. Intergenerational discrepancies of parental control among Chinese American families: links to family conflict and adolescent depressive symptoms. J Adolesc. 2007;30(6):965–75. http://dx.doi.org/10.1016/j.adolescence.2007.01.004.
91. Wu C, Chao RK. Intergenerational cultural conflicts in norms of parental warmth among Chinese American immigrants. Int J Behav Dev. 2005;29(6):516–23. doi:10.1177/01650250500147444.
92. Costigan CL, Dokis DP. Relations between parent-child acculturation differences and adjustment within immigrant Chinese families. Child Dev. 2006;77(5):1252–67. doi:10.1111/j.1467-8624.2006.00932.x.
93. Lau AS, McCabe KM, Yeh M, Garland AF, Wood PA, Hough RL. The acculturation gap-distress hypothesis among high-risk Mexican American families. J Fam Psychol. 2005;19(3):367–75. doi:10.1037/0893-3200.19.3.367.
94. Telzer EH. Expanding the acculturation gap-distress model: an integrative review of research. Hum Dev. 2010;53(6):313–40. doi:10.1159/000322476.
95. Juang LP, Syed M. Family cultural socialization practices and ethnic identity among college-going emerging adults. J Adolesc. 2010;33(3):347–54. doi:10.1016/j.adolescence.2009.11.008.
96. Lee R. Resilience against discrimination: ethnic identity and other-group orientation as protective factors for Korean Americans. J Couns Psychol. 2005;52:36–44.
97. Juang L, Nguyen, HH. Acculturation and adjustment in Asian American children and families. In Leong FT, Juang L, Qin DB, Fitzgerald HE, editors. Asian American and Pacifica Islander children and mental health, vol. 1. Santa Barbara, CA: ABC-CLIO, LLC; 2011. p. 71–96.
98. Kiang L, Yip T, Gonzales-Backen M, Witkow M, Fuligni AJ. Ethnic identity and the daily psychological well-being of adolescents from Mexican and Chinese backgrounds. Child Dev. 2006;77:1338–50. doi:10.1111/j.1467- 8624.2006.00938.x.
99. Lee R. Do ethnic identity and other-group orientation protect against discrimination for Asian Americans? J Couns Psychol. 2003;50:133–41.

100. Lee R, Yoo HC. Structure and measurement of ethnic identity for Asian American college students. J Couns Psych. 2004; 51(2): 263-69.
101. Umana-Taylor, AJ, Diversi, M, Fine, MA. Ethnic diversity and self-esteem of Latino adolescents: Distinctions among the Latino populations. Journal of Adolescent Research. 2002; 17(3):303-27. doi:10.1177/0743558402173005.
102. Chen C, Greenberger E, Lester J, Dong Q, Guo M-S. A cross-cultural study of family and peer correlates of adolescent misconduct. Dev Psychol. 1998;34(4):770–81. doi:10.1037/0012-1649.34.4.770.
103. Fuligni AJ. Authority, autonomy, and parent–adolescent conflict and cohesion: a study of adolescents from Mexican, Chinese, Filipino, and European backgrounds. Dev Psychol. 1998;34(4):782–92. doi:10.1037/0012-1649.34.4.782.
104. Greenberger E, Chen C. Perceived family relationships and depressed mood in early and late adolescence: a comparison of European and Asian Americans. Dev Psychol. 1996;32(4):707–16. doi:10.1037/0012-1649.32.4.707.
105. Laursen B, Coy KC, Collins WA. Reconsidering changes in parent–child conflict across adolescence: a meta-analysis. Child Dev. 1998;69(3):817–32. doi:10.2307/1132206.
106. Smetana JG. Culture, autonomy, and personal jurisdiction in adolescent-parent relationships. In: Kail RV, Reese HW, editors. Advances in child development and behavior, vol. 29. San Diego, CA: Academic; 2002. p. 51–87.
107. Steinberg L, Morris AS. Adolescent development. Annu Rev Psychol. 2001;52:83–110. doi:10.1146/annurev.psych.52.1.83.
108. Yau J, Smetana JG. Adolescent–parent conflict among Chinese adolescents in Hong Kong. Child Dev. 1996;67(3):1262–75. doi:10.2307/1131891.
109. Juang LP, Syed M, Cookston JT, Wang Y, Kim SY. Acculturation-based and everyday family conflict in Chinese American families. In: Juang LP, Umaña-Taylor AJ, editors. Family conflict among Chinese- and Mexican-origin adolescents and their parents in the U.S., vol. 2012. San Francisco, CA: Jossey-Bass; 2012. p. 13–34.
110. Kang H, Okazaki S, Abelmann N, Kim-Prieto C, Shanshan L. Redeeming immigrant parents: how Korean American emerging adults reinterpret their childhood. J Adolesc Res. 2010;25(3):441–64. doi:10.1177/0743558410361371.
111. Szapocznik J, Rio A, Perez-Vidal A, Kurtines W, Hervis O, Santisteban D. Bicultural effectiveness training (BET): an experimental test of an intervention modality for families experiencing intergenerational/intercultural conflict. Hisp J Behav Sci. 1986;8(4):303–30. doi:10.1177/07399863860084001.
112. Szapocznik J, Kurtines WM. Family psychology and cultural diversity: opportunities for theory, research, and application. In: Rule-Goldberger N, Bennet-Veroff J, editors. Annual convention of the American psychological association. New York, NY: New York University Press; 1995. p. 808–24.
113. Ying Y-W. Strengthening Intergenerational/Intercultural Ties in Immigrant Families (SITIF): a parenting intervention to bridge the Chinese American intergenerational acculturation gap. In: Trinh N-H, Rho YC, Lu FG, Sanders KM, Trinh N-H, Rho YC, Lu FG, Sanders KM, editors. Handbook of mental health and acculturation in Asian American families. Totowa, NJ: Humana; 2009. p. 45–64.
114. Ying Y-W. Strengthening intergenerational/intercultural ties in migrant families: a new intervention for parents. J Commun Psychol. 1999;27(1):89–96. doi:10.1002/(SICI)1520-6629(199901)27:1<89::AID-JCOP6>3.0.CO;2-O.
115. Falicov CJ. Latino families in therapy. New York, NY: Guilford; 2014.
116. McBrien JL. Educational needs and barriers for refugee students in the United States: a review of the literature. Rev Educ Res. 2005;75(3):329–64. doi:10.3102/00346543075003329.
117. Walsh F. Strengthening family resilience. 2nd ed. New York, NY: Guilford; 2006.
118. Golby BJ, Bretherton I. Resilience in postdivorce mother-child relationships. In: McCubbin HI, Thompson EA, Thomspson AI, Futrell JA, editors. The dynamics of resilient families. Thousand Oaks, CA: Sage; 1999. p. 237–69.

119. Amatea ES, Smith-Adcock S, Villares E. From family deficit to family strength: viewing families' contributions to children's learning from a family resilience perspective. Prof Sch Couns. 2006;9(3):177–89.
120. Szapocznik J, Kurtines W, Santisteban DA, Pantin H. The evolution of structural ecosystemic theory for working with Latino families. In: García JG, Zea MC, editors. Psychological interventions and research with Latino populations. Needham Heights, MA: Allyn & Bacon; 1997. p. 166–90.
121. Walsh F. Traumatic loss and major disasters: strengthening family and community resilience. Fam Process. 2007;46(2):207–27. doi:10.1111/j.1545-5300.2007.00205.x.
122. Rumbault RG. Profiles in resilience: educational achievement and ambition among children of immigrants in Southern California. In: Taylor RD, Wang MC, editors. Resilience across contexts: family, work, culture, and community. Mahwah, NY: Lawrence Erlbaum; 2000. p. 257–94.
123. Leong F, Part YS, Kalibatseva Z. Disentangling immigrant status in mental health: psychological protective and risk factors among Latino and Asian American immigrants. Am J Orthopsychiatry. 2013;83(2.3):361–71. doi:10.1111/ajop.12020.
124. Leidy ML, Guerra NG, Toro RI. Positive parenting, family cohesion, and child social competence among immigrant Latino families. J Latina/o Psychol. 2012;1(S):3–13. doi:10.1037/2168-1678.1.S.3.
125. Xia YR, Zhou ZG, Xie Z. Strengths and resilience in Chinese immigrant families: an initial effort of inquiry. In: Bengtson VL, Acock AC, Allen KR, Dilworth-Anderson P, Klein DM, editors. Sourcebook of family theory and research. Thousand Oaks, CA: Sage; 2005. p. 108–11.
126. Usita PM, Blieszner R. Immigrant family strengths: meeting communication challenges. J Fam Issues. 2002;23(2):266–86. doi:10.1177/0192513X02023002005.
127. Ayón C, Bou Ghosn Naddy M. Latino immigrant families' social support networks: strengths and limitations during time of stringent immigration legislation and economic insecurity. J Commun Psychol. 2013;41(3):359–77. doi:10.1002/jcop.21542.123.
128. Puyat JH. Is the influence of social support on mental health the same for immigrants and non-immigrants? J Immigr Minor Health. 2013;15:598–605. doi:10.1007/s10903-012-9658-7.124.
129. Hurtado-de-Mendoza A, Gonzales FA, Serrano A, Kaltman S. Social isolation and perceived barriers to establishing social networks among Latino immigrants. Am J Community Psychol. 2014;53(1):73–82. doi:10.1007/s10464-013-9619-x.125.
130. Ashborne LM, Baobaid M, Azizova KS. Expanding notions of family time and parental monitoring: parents' and adolescents' experiences of time spent together and apart in Muslim immigrant families. J Comp Fam Stud. 2012;43(2):201–15.

School-Based Interventions

Alisa B. Miller, Colleen B. Bixby, and B. Heidi Ellis

Abstract

In this chapter, we provide a brief history of school-based interventions, the connection between mental health and academics, and the provision of school-based mental health services, with a specific focus on immigrant youth. Immigrant youth within the US school system are described, as well as considerations in delivering mental health services to them within the school context. Various approaches to interventions (i.e., universal, selected, and indicated) are reviewed. Case examples of interventions with good outcomes and effectiveness are showcased and professionals within a school system potentially involved in service provision are highlighted. Evaluation and sustainability of school-based mental health interventions are also discussed.

Keywords

Immigrant • School-based interventions • Youth • Children • Students • Mental health interventions • Schools • Service provision • Refugee

History of School-Based Interventions

There is a long history of clinicians working together with schools to improve the well-being of students [1, 2]. The relationship between schools and mental health services in the USA, however, is one that has been long and complex and has ebbed and flowed since the establishment of psychological clinics by academic/medical

A.B. Miller, Ph.D. (✉) • B.H. Ellis, Ph.D.
Department of Psychiatry, Boston Children's Hospital\Harvard Medical School,
300 Longwood Avenue, Boston, MA 02115, USA
e-mail: alisa.miller@childrens.harvard.edu

C. B. Bixby, M.P.H.
Department of Psychiatry, Boston Children's Hospital, Boston, MA, USA

© Springer International Publishing Switzerland 2016
S.G. Patel, D. Reicherter (eds.), *Psychotherapy for Immigrant Youth*,
DOI 10.1007/978-3-319-24693-2_4

Table 1 US historical sociocultural movements and corresponding mental health development in the school setting

Sociocultural movement	Mental health expansion
Community mental health movement after WWII	Schools viewed as appropriate community-based sites for mental health services
Civil Rights Movement of the 1960s	Legislation established that prohibited discrimination against and provided services to those with mental disabilities
Change in social mores from the 1960s through the 1980s	Increased student involvement in risky behaviors and pressure on schools to provide prevention/intervention services
School-based health clinic movement of the 1990s	Recognition of high prevalence of mental health issues in students and need for services

institutions in partnership with public schools in the 1890s [1]. Five historical sociocultural movements in the USA have been identified that all contributed to more awareness of student mental health and the corresponding need for the provision of mental health services in schools [2] (see Table 1). In addition, Sedlak [1] provides a historical perspective on the relationship between the schools and mental health services focusing on different aspects (e.g., service goals, professional roles, funding, etc.) that have presented challenges to this partnership.

Mental Health and Academics

Research on the relationship between mental health and achievement consistently reports that, as compared to youth without mental health problems, youth with mental health problems have lower school performance and attain lower levels of education [3]. Psychological distress may impact a student's ability to pay attention, hinder his or her executive functioning, and interfere with building social relationships among other areas important to immigrant youth. Roeser et al. [4] summarize data on the relationship between a child's emotional distress and achievement; students with internalized distress (e.g., sadness, anxiety, depression) show diminished academic functioning and those with externalized distress (e.g., anger, frustration) show school difficulties including learning delays and poor achievement. Longitudinal research has found that a student's increase in sadness or hopelessness was related to a subsequent decrease or lack of improvement in test scores in reading, language, and mathematics [5]. Hanson et al. [5] also showed that "beneficial influences" or in other words protective factors such as caring relationships in school, high expectations at school, and meaningful community participation were related to increases in test scores. Poor academic performance and inconsistent attendance have been shown to be early signs of emerging mental health problems or of problems that already exist [6]. It has also been demonstrated that over half of adolescents who do not finish high school have a diagnosable psychiatric illness [7]. Of note, immigrant youth and children of immigrants are much less likely to graduate from high school than those children of US born parents, which may be attributable to high rates of poverty and high proportions of parents who did not graduate high school [8, 9].

Immigrant Youth in the School System

Immigrant students are the fastest-growing sector of students in the USA [10], as more and more parents settle here seeking a better future for themselves and their children [9, 11]. Taken together these data underscore the demographic shift occurring in the USA and resulting change in the school landscape. It also highlights the need for schools to be able to respond to the unique needs of their immigrant student population.

Mental Health Interventions in the School Setting

The continued efforts to implement mental health interventions in the school setting derive in large part from the recognition that students with mental health issues have more school difficulties (e.g., school expulsions, absenteeism, etc.) and have poorer outcomes (e.g., lower graduation rates) than those without [3, 12] and that traditional mental health services are underutilized by youth [13]. It has been demonstrated that ethnic minority, youth in particular, underutilize mental health services [13–15] as well as immigrant and refugee youth [16–18]. In addition, research has also shown that limited English proficiency (LEP) is one of the most powerful predictors of lower use of mental health services [19].

When youth do utilize services, it is oftentimes in the school setting [20, 21]. Thus, schools and educators have much to gain from students receiving appropriate mental health treatment because when mental health needs go unaddressed, academic performance suffers. At the same time, mental health practitioners recognize that offering school-based interventions holds the potential to address both mental health barriers to academic success and structural barriers to youth accessing mental health services. This is particularly relevant for schools with immigrant students given that immigrant students account for growing numbers in the US school system, present with unique mental health needs, and have higher high school dropout rates than US born youth.

Despite the many advantages of school-based mental health services, successful implementation of these services faces a number of challenges [22, 23]. There are standard challenges such as funding concerns, lack of adequately trained mental health school-based professionals, and lack of school administrator or staff buy-in [22, 23] that impact the implementation of school-based mental health programs. Two educational policies also shape the landscape in which school-based mental health programs operate: (1) the Individuals with Disabilities Education Act (IDEA) of 1994 (reauthorization in 2004) and (2) the No Child Left Behind Act (NCLB) in 2002. (For a more comprehensive history of education policy and its interface with mental health, please see Kataoka et al. [12].) In addition, the implementation of school-based mental health programs with immigrants faces its own unique challenges. The remainder of this chapter focuses on school-based mental health interventions that address the unique challenges and needs of immigrant and refugee youth.

Considerations in Delivering Mental Health Services to Immigrant Youth

We highlight here several considerations in implementing school-based mental health services with immigrants: heterogeneity of immigrant populations, confidentiality, family involvement, and the importance of the socio-ecological framework. Immigrant youth and families represent a multitude of different backgrounds and experiences including reasons for migration, experience of migration, languages, and cultures. This heterogeneity can prove challenging to schools, as youth and their families vary in the amount and types of mental health support they need to make a successful transition to school and the community. In addition, there is a large need to service the variety of languages spoken by immigrant families but a shortage of translators and limited language and cultural resources available to schools to help communicate with youth and families. Schools are challenged to have the cultural and linguistic capacity needed to keep up with the increasing numbers of immigrant youth, and there is a real need to provide adequate culturally appropriate training of school personnel to attend to immigrant youth and their families [24, 25].

An important consideration when delivering mental health services to an immigrant population is keeping confidentiality. Confidentiality is of particular concern both within the school setting and within ethnic communities. It is mandated in mental health services so that one's personal information cannot be shared without permission [22]. Issues of confidentiality become particularly salient in immigrant communities where there is stigma around mental health and mental health services [26]. Relatedly, legal issues must be considered when working with immigrant communities. For example, immigrants who have arrived in the USA without sufficient legal documentation or those in the midst of legal procedures related to immigration status may be less likely or worrisome to convey personal information to anyone at a public institution including a school. Given the tight-knit nature of some immigrant communities, some families may also fear that information about their child will be shared with other community members. This is prominent among immigrant communities where translators are often people from within the same community. The concern of private information being shared may also be increased or intensified for those who are representatives of more rare cultures/languages within a given community. Ellis and colleagues [26] assert that "in some instances, community members may be concerned that if a child is known to be receiving mental health care, the stigma he or she may experience would be more damaging than receiving no care at all" (p. 71). Thus extra care must be taken to ensure confidentiality. This is especially true in a school setting where students may be aware of when another student is being pulled out of a class for services. A balance must be struck between sharing student information in the service of improvement or student success, sharing clinical information about a student (e.g., safety concerns), and sharing information about the youth that does not need to be shared within the school or with others in the immigrant community [22, 26].

Another consideration for service delivery with immigrant youth is family engagement, both with the school system in general and with mental health services. Immigrant parents may have varying knowledge of the US school system or of schooling in general [27] or at times due in part to their own lack of educational attainment. Even if they are familiar with the institution of school, culturally they may have different expectations of the role of the school, the teachers, and/or themselves in their child's education [25]. These challenges to engage immigrant families in the school system can be compounded by the difficulty that immigrant children and families have in accessing mental health services, including the stigma of mental health across various cultural groups [11, 13, 28]. Although parents may be concerned with behaviors at home or in school, they may not understand the psychological sequelae to these behaviors [29]. This may reflect different cultural understandings of mental health issues [16]. Alternatively, these symptoms might be seen as less important relative to other factors; the acculturative stress experience by immigrant families may have more prominence in daily life as they struggle to meet their housing, healthcare, and employment needs [30]. Schools need to take these challenges into consideration in engaging immigrant families in the school system and mental health services.

Finally, when implementing mental health services, it also important to understand a youth's immigration experience from a socio-ecological framework [31]. Assessing a student within his or her individual, familial, societal, and cultural contexts is critical to addressing the mental health and overall well-being of immigrant youth [32–34]. These issues related to the socio-ecological context (e.g., ethnic identity, gender, trauma exposure, community violence, poverty, discrimination) can have an impact on the overall well-being of students, contributing to learning, socio-emotional, and behavioral problems [35, 36]. Pumariega and Rothe [18] provide a comprehensive overview of the unique challenges of immigration (e.g., migration experience, acculturative stressors, etc.) and discuss factors such as acculturation status that may minimize risk of poor mental health in immigrant youth. Of note, they report that the less acculturated an individual, the better his or her mental health profile; first-generation immigrants fare better than 1.5[1] or second-generation immigrants in terms of psychopathology [18]. Similarly, Ellis et al. [33] provide a thoughtful overview of the unique challenges of refugees and broaden the understanding of the refugee experience to include core stressors of trauma, resettlement, isolation, and acculturation.

Rationale for School-Based Mental Health Intervention

The school system is a promising setting to increase access to mental health services [37], particularly for immigrant youth [26, 38, 39]. Schools are uniquely poised to meet the aforementioned considerations for a few key reasons: schools are gateway

---

[1]The term 1.5 generation describe people who were born in another country and arrived in the USA as children and adolescents.

providers that allow for the engagement of immigrant youth and families, schools allow for early identification of mental health need among immigrant students, and school-based interventions can address the socio-ecological framework that is critical to these youth.

Stiffman and colleagues [40] describe how a child's mental health is determined by key individuals, or gateway providers, who both have the ability to influence decisions about help seeking and the information related to available resources. School-based staff (e.g., teachers, coaches, front desk administrators, etc.) represent gateway providers for immigrant youth and families since schools are a key part of the resettlement experience. Schools provide a shared and common context for those whose environments and experiences have been disrupted by trauma and displacement, such as refugee and immigrant youth. They are one of the earliest systems that are introduced in resettlement and are often highly respected institutions by these families. School-based staff can help parents navigate what is initially an unfamiliar school system and at the same time expose them to mental health services and resources available. As schools develop trust and relationships with these families, the process of referral or integration into mental health services is more easily facilitated. Schools therefore play a key role in decreasing the stigma of mental health services among immigrant populations [32, 41]. Finally, the transportation barriers that are endemic to the underutilization of mental health services (in clinic settings) by immigrant populations are not usually involved in accessing schools. This context of familiarity, de-stigmatization, and access becomes a unique opportunity to deliver mental health services to refugee and immigrant youth [41–43].

The school environment also provides for the early identification of immigrant youth in need of services. Teachers and auxiliary school staff have the unique perspective of being able to observe children in a number of different settings and activities during the school day, over different periods of time, and with different individuals such as other students, friends, and adults [44]. Teachers, school administrators, and other school staff are able to observe these children in a nonstigmatizing manner, providing information related to needed mental health services that might not be available otherwise.

Finally, school-based intervention has the potential to address the broader socio-ecological context that is critical to serving the mental health needs of immigrant youth. The process of acculturation, which often integrates multiple levels of the socio-ecological context, is a defining feature of an immigrant youth's experience [39, 45]. This process may be particularly prominent in the school setting as youth navigate daily intercultural interactions with their peers and teachers outside of their familial and cultural contexts. The combination of the process of acculturation with the developmental transition that these youth are going through makes them especially amenable to supportive interventions [42, 43]. It has therefore been suggested that the school context, where immigrant children are navigating acculturation and striving for overall adjustment, is the appropriate place to provide mental healthcare [46, 47]. Addressing acculturation as part of a mental health intervention can help how youth learn and how they relate to other students and youth [48]. Thus, school-based interventions are well positioned to provide timely mental health services that incorporate a focus on the broader social context that immigrant youth are experiencing.

Approaches to School-Based Mental Health Interventions

Schools can provide mental health services to immigrant youth through a number of different approaches. There are a number of practical considerations when designing school-based services such as the demographics of the population (ethnicity, age, and gender), the setting in which the school is located (i.e., urban vs. suburban), and when services will be offered (integrated as part of the regular academic curriculum, offered during electives, or held after school). For example, the demographics of the population will affect the curriculum/content being offered (e.g., boys versus girls) and whether any group services are mixed-group or a single ethnicity, gender, or grade level. Another example is the setting of the school and availability of transportation, which may impact how children get home or when services can be offered. Similarly, the timing of services during the school day will impact what other content the children will miss and how singled out they feel/appear to others when receiving services.

School-based mental health services vary, both in terms of focusing on prevention versus more acute intervention and also in terms of who provides these services (see below for a discussion of individuals involved in service provision). We adapted the following table from the American Academy of Pediatrics [22] to provide an overview of how a school or school district can configure mental health services using a three-tiered model of services [2, 22] (see Table 2). The configuration of services should depend upon the refugee or immigrant population in the school, the broader school population, existing mental health capacity in the school, and partnerships with agencies outside of the school. Multiple tiers of services can be combined into one program, along the lines of a public health prevention model that includes a spectrum of activities across different levels of prevention and intervention. Comprehensive services that address multiple layers of intervention may be the most successful for immigrant youth [49, 50], and schools are key settings to provide this range of prevention, early identification, and treatment [28, 44, 51].

Table 2 Overview of school-based services, targeted participants, and overall focus of intervention

Services	Target participants	Overall focus
Universal services: preventive mental health programs and services	All children in all school settings	Decrease risk factors (e.g., risk-taking behaviors) and build resilience (e.g., school connectedness)
Selected services: group or individual therapy	Students who have identified mental health needs or risks	Individual students' identified emotional or behavioral issues
Indicated services: multidisciplinary team services including but not limited to special education services, individual and family therapy, pharmacotherapy, and school and social agency coordination	Students with mental health diagnoses	Individual students' identified needs in multiple areas of functioning

A universal intervention is delivered to the whole school or classroom and usually involves a transformation of the school environment as opposed to implementation of a specific treatment modality. One of the most common types of a school-based mental health universal intervention is social and emotional learning (SEL) that focuses on the relationship between social and emotional competencies, the development of character, and a core set of life principles and academic achievement [52]. Durlak et al. [48] did a meta-analysis of 213 school-based, universal SEL programs and found that these programs improved socio-emotional competencies, attitudes, academic performance, and pro-social behaviors [48]. SEL programs have been adapted for Latino immigrant populations with favorable results [53]. Another example is the Cultural Adjustment and Trauma Services (CATS) model, a comprehensive program for first- and second-generation immigrant children with significant trauma exposure and/or cultural adjustment needs [46]. At the universal level, CATS provides relationship building between school personnel and immigrant students, coordination services aimed at reducing stress in the school environment, and supportive resources for families and outreach services [46]. A third example of a universal intervention is creative expression workshops that involve music, creative play, drama, and drawing. These workshops have been used to address general adjustment issues and have been shown to increase feelings of integration as well as decrease levels of emotional and behavioral symptoms [54].

Case Study

Project SHIFA (Supporting the Health of Immigrant Families and Adolescents), a multitiered model that involved a universal component, was developed to specifically address challenges to engaging Somali youth and families in services, as well as problems associated with traumatic stress [26, 55]. It was developed through a partnership between agencies with specific expertise in mental health, education, and Somali culture. Project SHIFA was based in a middle school in the Boston Public School District and provided secondary prevention and intervention services to Somali English language learner (ELL) middle school students and their families.

Project SHIFA is a four-tiered integrated and comprehensive model of prevention and intervention. Tier one is community outreach and engagement, which seeks to address the challenge of parent and community engagement as well as address the barrier of stigma around mental illness and treatment. Tier two is comprised of school-based nonclinical skill-building groups, which seeks to teach emotion regulation and coping skills as well as provide a safe space for youth to discuss acculturation issues. Stigma of services is reduced by inviting all Somali ELL students to join the groups. In addition, the groups provide a method for monitoring individual youth, which aids in the collection of diagnostic information, especially in reference to their peers, who may need more targeted or intensive services. Tier three is individual outpatient/ school-based therapy, which targets the specific needs of the child. Tier four is home-based therapy, which enables more intensive work with families. The evidence-based model implemented in Tiers three and four is trauma systems therapy (TST). TST is a treatment model that views the development of traumatic stress in children as resulting from two main elements: (1) a traumatized child who is not able to regulate emotional states and (2) a social environment or system of care that is not sufficiently able to help the child contain this dysregulation [56].

A lesson learned from the implementation of Project SHIFA, Boston, is that inclusivity and flexibility are key to engaging refugee families in a mental health program [57]. A clear example of the flexibility and responsiveness to the community needed in implementing a program in a refugee community is highlighted by the following. In Project SHIFA, Boston, community outreach and anti-stigma efforts, in combination with parent engagement during the time their children participated in the school-based groups, resulted in exceptionally high success rate with referrals for individual and family mental health services. As school was not viewed as a comfortable, accessible place for some families to meet with clinicians, Project SHIFA partnered with a home-based agency to provide in-home services.

Selected school-based interventions for immigrant youth are designed to target mental health symptoms more directly and are delivered to those who have been identified as at risk for or as having mental health needs. Selected interventions for immigrant youth have the goal of preventing and/or improving functioning and often employ therapeutic components eclectically rather than as part of a structured protocol. Selected interventions for immigrant youth are often delivered as part of a multitiered program that incorporates universal and/or targeted services. An example of a selected mental health intervention is one tier of the aforementioned CATS program. Supportive therapy, psychoeducation, and cognitive behavioral therapy (CBT) techniques are provided to a subset of the immigrant children in response to clinical presentation and/or cultural adjustment needs [46].

Targeted school-based interventions for immigrant youth focus on populations with a specific diagnosis. These interventions usually involve a therapeutic component focused on the verbal processing of past experiences and are often targeted toward PTSD or depression. The CATS program employed trauma-focused CBT (TF-CBT) to treat children with PTSD or if they identified a specific traumatic event as related to their current problems [46]. A second example of a targeted intervention for immigrant youth is Cognitive Behavioral Intervention for Trauma in Schools (CBITS) [38, 58]. CBITS was designed for a multicultural population in an inner city school in response to community violence exposure. CBITS has since been adapted for American Indian adolescents who presented with symptoms of PTSD and depression [38, 59]. CBITS is comprised of teacher psychoeducation, a 10-week CBT group therapy (focused on anxiety, PTSD, and depression symptoms), as well as individual youth and optional parent sessions [59]. Finally, the Mental Health for Immigrants Program (MHIP) [38] is based on the CBITS program and is offered to newly immigrated Latino children. Youth who screened positive for exposure to violence and clinically significant symptoms of PTSD and/or depression received eight sessions of CBT group therapy.

The aforementioned universal, selected, and targeted school-based interventions have been effective with the specific populations for which they were developed. In some cases, i.e., CBITS with Latino children, as well as (nonimmigrant) Native American Indian adolescents, the intervention has been adapted for multiple populations with success [38, 59]. A review of the literature shows a lack of school-based interventions that have been used with multiple populations, especially with various cultural groups; the approach has been to demonstrate effectiveness with one group. The next step would be to determine if the principles of the intervention are generalizable to other cultural or ethnic populations. In the case of TST-R (the in-depth case study above), the intervention was developed and evaluated with Somali refugee youth and is currently being implemented and evaluated with Bhutanese refugee youth, with considerations for expanding the model to mixed-ethnicity groups (M. A. Benson, personal communication, May 20, 2015).

Individuals Involved in the Provision of School-Based Mental Health Services

Given the limited resources and high demand for provision of mental health services in the school setting, clinicians should be prepared to work in collaboration with existing school resources and personnel [60]. According to the *National Association of School Psychologists* (www.nasponline.org), most school-based mental health services will be provided by school-employed professionals such as guidance counselors, psychologists, and social workers. These professionals will have training in learning and mental health within the school context and can contribute to academic and school success. Community-employed professionals also may provide mental health services in schools and/or across school districts through intra-agency agreements. In this case, mental health providers from the community agency deliver services within the school setting. These professionals usually focus on the global mental health of students and how it impacts the students' functioning in the contexts of family, community, and work. The AAP [22] also offers a way to understand the various mental health service delivery models that are utilized by schools or school districts (see Table 3). The identified models and model components are not exclusive and schools may offer one or more components of these models [22].

Given the increasing numbers of immigrant students in the school system, it is important for schools, teachers, and other school staff to provide culturally and linguistically appropriate services in response to the needs of their immigrant

Table 3 Mental health models and corresponding model components

Mental health model	Components of model

School supported	Providers are employees of the school system:
	  Social workers
	  Guidance counselors
	  School psychologists
	Separate mental health units exist within the school system
	School nurses serve as a major portal of entry for students with mental health concerns

Community connected	A mental health agency or individual delivers direct services in the school part time or full time under contract Mental health professionals are available within a school-based health center or are invited into after-school programs Formal linkage to an off-site mental health professional and/or to a managed care organization
Comprehensive, integrated	A comprehensive and integrated mental health program addresses prevention strategies, school environment, screening, referral, special education, and family and community issues and delivers direct mental health services School-based health clinics provide comprehensive and integrated health and mental health services within the school environment

students and families. As such, in the process of implementing a school-based mental health program with immigrant youth, it would be beneficial to provide on-going professional development opportunities to teachers and school staff [23, 61] across varying domains relevant to the provision of services and mental health of immigrant students (e.g., evidence-based interventions, emotion science, reasons for migration, etc.). It has been recommended, however, that professional development opportunities should not be prescribed or regulated but that a more flexible approach be taken [61]. An approach that is responsive to the needs of the school, the teachers themselves, as well as the needs of the students [61].

Evaluation

Evaluation of school-based mental health programs for immigrant youth is important, as the research base for what is known to be effective for these populations is limited. As part of this evaluation, outcomes must be measured in order for an intervention to be considered either efficacious or effective. Efficacy is defined by how well an intervention performs under ideal and controlled conditions, such as in an academic research center, whereas effectiveness is defined by how well an intervention performs under real-world conditions like in a school context [60]. Outcome targets of interest may differ for different stakeholders such as schools, parents, and mental health systems. As such, it is important to define what is meaningful when considering evaluation or outcome measures [60]. It may be beneficial for program evaluators to consider what outcomes may be meaningful to different stakeholders such as school administrators (e.g., attendance, GPA, standardized test scores, graduation rates), teachers (e.g., reductions in stress, opportunities for professional trainings), students (e.g., increased sense of school belonging, acculturation), parents (e.g., academic performance, reduced disciplinary measures), and the researcher/clinician (e.g., improvement in mental health symptoms). Program evaluation is not only essential to demonstrate a program's effectiveness but also can provide invaluable information about the quality and perceived value of the program. The collection of outcome data can lead to improved and meaningful outcomes for participants and may also be leveraged to obtain funding for the program in the future [60].

Sustainability

Once a school-based mental health program for immigrant youth has been developed, implemented, and shown to be effective, the question turns to how to sustain or maintain it. In addition to the standard barrier of funding, sustaining school-based mental health programs for immigrant youth involves the unique challenge of obtaining buy-in from multiple stakeholders, including school and community. Integration of services within the school context is crucial to gaining school administrator and staff buy-in, but the program must also be flexible and responsive to the needs of the community it serves. Just as it is paramount that school administrators and staff view mental health services as not only worthwhile but also critical to the well-being and adjustment of their immigrant students, it is also paramount for the immigrant community. One means of accomplishing this may be making explicit the connections between mental health services, improved academic success, and increased parent engagement to school administration and staff and creating a mechanism of providing positive feedback to immigrant parents. Another may be to provide professional development opportunities to teachers and school staff on topics integral to the program (e.g., cultural presentations of the targeted ethnic community, presentation of the consequences of mental health disorders like PTSD on academic learning in youth, etc.). It may also be beneficial to offer needed or desired services to immigrant parents in the school setting (e.g., English as a second language class, navigating the US school system 101, etc.). Activities such as these contribute to program ownership by and engagement of key stakeholders [26, 55].

In addition, the development of school-based mental health intervention in consultation and collaboration with key partners like community leaders, parents, and the school is critical for sustainability [10, 26]. Partnership with the community is essential to develop a school-based mental health program that is consistent with community needs, priorities, values, and culture [26, 62]. Partnership with the school is critical to cultivate buy-in and accountability as well as to address practical issues of implementing services such as space and time and obtaining consent [22]. It has also been recommended that interventions be grounded in strength-based approaches [10] that acknowledge, leverage, and view as an asset the diverse cultural factors of immigrant communities.

Conclusion

Immigrant youth represent an increasing population in US schools. In order to best service these students, we must be able to attend to their overall well-being and adjustment to the USA, which may include responding to their socio-emotional needs. Schools are uniquely poised to deliver mental health services to refugee and immigrant youth, as they address structural barriers to accessing mental health services. Embedding culturally appropriate mental health services in the school provides an invaluable opportunity to overcome mental health barriers in order to promote academic and life success of immigrant youth in the USA.

References

1. Sedlak MW. The uneasy alliance of mental health services and the schools: an historical perspective. Am J Orthopsychiatry. 1997;67:349–62. doi:10.1037/h0080238.
2. Walter HJ. School-based interventions. In: Wiener J, Dulcan M, editors. Dulcan's textbook of child and adolescent psychiatry. Arlington, VA: American Psychiatric Publishing; 2009.
3. McLeod JD, Fettes DL. Trajectories of failure: the educational careers of children with mental health problems. Am J Sociol. 2007;113(3):653–701. doi:10.1086/521849.
4. Roeser RW, Eccles JS, Strobel KR. Linking the study of schooling and mental health: selected issues and empirical illustrations at the level of the individual. Educ Psychol. 1998;33:153–76. doi:10.1207/s15326985ep3304_2.
5. Hanson TL, Austin G, Lee-Bayha J. Ensuring that No Child Is Left Behind: how are student health risks & resilience related to the academic progress of schools? San Francisco, CA: WestEd, Health and Human Development Program; 2004. Available at https://chks.wested.org/resources/EnsuringNCLB.pdf.
6. DeSocio J, Hootman J. Children's mental health and school success. Journal of School Nursing. 2004;20(4):189–96. doi:10.1177/10598405040200040201.
7. Vander Stoep A, Weiss N, Kuo E, Cheney D, Cohen P. What proportion of failure to complete secondary school in the US population is attributable to adolescent psychiatric disorder? J Behav Health Serv Res. 2003;30(1):119–24. doi:10.1007/BF02287817.
8. Child Trends. Child trends' calculations of U.S. Census Bureau, school enrollment--social and economic characteristics of students: October 2005: Detailed Tables: Table 1; 2005. http://www.census.gov/population/www/socdemo/school/cps2005.html. Retrieved from http://www.childtrendsdatabank.org/pdf/1_PDF.pdf
9. Hernandez DJ, Napierala JS. Children in immigrant families: essential to America's future. Foundation for Child Development: Child and Youth Well-Being Index Policy Brief; 2012.
10. Bal A, Perzigian ABT. Evidence-based interventions for immigrant students experiencing behavioral and academic problems: a systematic review of the literature. Educ Treat Child. 2013;36(4):5–28. doi:10.1353/etc.2013.0044.
11. Hernandez DJ. Demographic change and the life circumstances of immigrant families. Futur Child. 2004;14(2):17–47. doi:10.2307/1602792. Available at: http://futureofchildren.org/futureofchildren/publications/docs/14_02_2.pdf.
12. Kataoka SH, Rowan B, Hoagwood KE. Bridging the divide: In search of common ground in mental health and education. Res Policy. 2009;60(11):1510–5. doi:10.1176/ps.2009.60.11.1510.
13. Kataoka SH, Zhang L, Wells KB. UnmetnNeed for mental health care among U.S. children: variation by ethnicity and insurance status. Am J Psychiatr. 2002;159(9):1548–55. doi:10.1176/appi.ajp.159.9.1548.
14. Coard S, Holden E. The effect of racial and ethnic diversity on the delivery of mental health services in pediatric primary care. J Clin Psychol Med Settings. 1998;5(3):275–94. doi:10.1023/A:1026202103101.

15. Howard M, Hodes M. Psychopathology, adversity, and service utilization of young refugees. J Am Acad Child Adolesc Psychiatry. 2000;39(3):368–77. doi:10.1097/00004583-200003000-00020.
16. Ellis BH, Lincoln AK, Charney ME, Ford-Paz R, Benson M, Strunin L. Mental health service utilization of Somali adolescents: religion, community, and school as gateways to healing. Transcult Psychiatry. 2010;47(5):789–811. doi:10.1177/1363461510379933.
17. Lustig S, Kia-Keating M, Knight WG, Geltman P, Ellis BH, Kinzie JD, Keane T, Saxe G. Review of child and adolescent refugee mental health. J Am Acad Child Adolesc Psychiatry. 2004;43(1):24–36.
18. Pumariega AJ, Rothe E. Leaving no children or families outside: the challenges of immigration. Am J Orthopsychiatry. 2010;80(4):505–15. doi:10.1111/j.1939-0025.2010.01053.x.
19. Sentell T, Shumway M, Snowden LJ. Access to mental health treatment by English language proficiency and race/ethnicity. J Gen Intern Med. 2007;22(2):289–93. doi:10.1007/s11606-007-0345-7.
20. Stephan SH, Weist M, Kataoka S, Adelsheim S, Mills C. Transformation of children's mental health services: the role of school mental health. Psychiatr Serv. 2007;58:1330–8. doi:10.1176/appi.ps.58.10.1330.
21. Williams JH, Horvath VE, Wei HS, Van DRA, Jonson RM. Teachers' perspectives of children's mental health service needs in urban elementary schools. Child Sch. 2007;29:95–106. doi:10.1093/cs/29.2.95.
22. American Academy of Pediatrics. Committee on school based mental health. School-Based Mental Health Services. Pediatrics. 2004;113(6):1839–45. doi:10.1542/peds.2009-1415.
23. Macklem GL. The challenge of providing mental health services in schools. In: Macklem GL, editor. Evidence-based school mental health services. New York: Springer; 2011. p. 1–17. Available at: http://dx.doi.org/10.1007/978-1-4419-7907-0_1.
24. Trumbull E, Rothstein-Fisch C, Greenfield PM. Bridging cultures in our schools: new approaches that work. Knowledge Brief; 2000.
25. Trumbull E, Rothstein-Fisch C, Greenfield P, Quiroz B. Bridging culture between home and school: a guide for teachers. Mahwah, NJ: Lawrence Erlbaum; 2001.
26. Ellis BH, Miller AB, Baldwin H, Abdi S. New directions in refugee youth mental health services: overcoming barriers to engagement. J Child Adolesc Trauma. 2011;4:69–85. doi:10.1080/19361521.2011.545047.
27. Carreon GP, Drake C, Barton AC. The importance of presence: immigrant parents' school engagement experiences. Am Educ Res J. 2005;42:465–98. doi:10.3102/00028312042003465.
28. Huang L, Stroul B, Friedman R, Mrazek P, Friesen B, Pires S, Mayberg S. Transforming mental health care for children and their families. Am Psychol. 2005;60(6):615–27. doi:10.1037/0003-066X.60.6.615.
29. Garrison EG, Roy IS, Azar V. Responding to the mental health needs of Latino children and families through school-based services. Clin Psychol Rev. 1999;19(2):199–219. doi:10.1016/S0272-7358(98)00070-1.
30. Westermeyer J, Wahmanholm K. Refugee children. In: Apfel RJ, Simon B, editors. Minefields in their hearts: the mental health of children in war and communal violence. New Haven, CT: Yale University Press; 1996. p. 75–103.
31. Bronfenbrenner U, Ceci SJ. Nature-nurture reconceptualized in developmental perspective: a biological model. Psychol Rev. 1994;101:568–86. doi:10.1037/h0044895.
32. American Psychological Association, Presidential Task Force on Immigration. Crossroads: The psychology of immigration in the new century; 2012. Retrieved from http://www.apa.org/topics/immigration/report.aspx
33. Ellis BH, Murray K, Barrett C. Understanding the mental health of refugees: trauma, stress, and the cultural context. In: Parekh R, editor. The Massachusetts general hospital textbook on diversity and cultural sensitivity in mental health. Current Clinical Psychiatry. New York: Humana; 2014. p. 165–87. doi:10.1007/978-1-4614-8918-4.
34. Murray KE, Davidson GR, Schweitzer RD. Review of refugee mental health interventions following resettlement: best practices and recommendations. Am J Orthopsychiatry. 2010;80(4):576–85. doi:10.1111/j.1939-0025.2010.01062.x.

35. Qin D. Being 'good' or being 'popular': gender and ethnic identity negotiations of Chinese immigrant adolescents. J Adolesc Res. 2009;24:37–66. doi:10.1177/0743558408326912.
36. Suarez-Orozco C, Rhodes J, Milburn M. Unraveling the immigrant paradox: academic engagement and disengagement among recently arrived immigrant youth. Youth and Society. 2009;41:151–85. doi:10.1177/0044118X09333647.
37. Allensworth D, Lawson E, Nicholson L, Wyche J. School and health: our nations investment. Washington, DC: National Academy; 1997.
38. Kataoka SH, Stein BD, Jaycox LH, Wong M, Escudero P, Tu W, et al. A school-based mental health program for traumatized Latino immigrant children. J Am Acad Adolesc Psychiatry. 2003;42:311–8. doi:10.1097/00004583-200303000-00011.
39. Tyrer RA, Fazel M. School and community-based interventions for refugee and asylum seeking children: a systematic review. PLoS One. 2014;9(2), e89359. doi:10.1371/journal. pone.0089359.
40. Stiffman AR, Pescosolido B, Cabassa LJ. Building a model to understand youth service access: the gateway provider model. Ment Health Serv Res. 2004;6(4):189–98. doi:10.1177/1363461510379933.
41. Rousseau C, Guzder J. School-based prevention programs for refugee children. Child Adolesc Psychiatr Clin N Am. 2008;17(3):533–49. doi:10.1016/j.chc.2008.02.002.
42. Hodes M, Jagdev D, Chandra N, Cunniff A. Risk and resilience for psychological distress amongst unaccompanied asylum seeking adolescents. J Child Psychol Psychiatry. 2008;49(7):723–32. doi:10.1111/j.1469-7610.2008.01912.x.
43. Jordans MD, Tol WA, Komproe IH, Susanty D, Vallipuram A, Ntamatumba P, et al. Development of a multi-layered psychosocial care system for children in areas of political violence. International Journal of Mental Health Systems. 2010;4:15. doi:10.1186/1752-4458-4-15.
44. Masia-Warner C, Nangle DW, Hansen DJ. Bringing evidence-based child mental health services to the schools: general issues and specific populations. Educ Treat Children. 2006;29(2):165–72.
45. Birman D, Chan WY. Screening and assessing immigrant and refugee youth in school-based mental health programs. Washington, DC: Center for Health and Health Care in Schools, The George Washington University; 2008. Retrieved from http://www.healthinschools.org/ Immigrant-and-Refugee-Children/%7E/media/55F5B8709C7D4AEBA06A42BFD0A9C B9B.ashx.
46. Beehler S, Birman D, Campbell R. The effectiveness of cultural adjustment and trauma services (CATS): generating practice-cased evidence on a comprehensive, school-based mental health intervention for immigrant youth. Am J Community Psychol. 2012;50(1):155–68. doi:10.1007/s10464-011-9486-2.
47. Birman D, Weinstein T, Chan W, Beehler S. Immigrant youth in U.S. schools: opportunities for prevention. Prev Res. 2007;14:14–7.
48. Durlak JA, Weissberg RP, Dymnicki AB, Taylor RD, Schellinger KB. The impact of enhancing students' social and emotional learning: a meta-analysis of school-based universal interventions. Child Dev. 2011;82:405–28. doi:10.1111/j.1467-8624.2010.01564.
49. Birman D, Beehler S, Harris EM, Everson ML, Batia K, Liautaud J, et al. International Family, Adult, and Child Enhancement Services (FACES): a community-based comprehensive services model for refugee children in resettlement. Am J Orthopsychiatry. 2008;78(1):121. doi:10.1037/0002-9432.78.1.121.
50. Birman D, Ho J, Pulley E, Batia K, Everson ML, Ellis H, et al. Mental health interventions for refugee children in resettlement: White Paper II from the National Child Traumatic Stress Network Refugee Trauma Task Force. Chicago: International FACES, Heartland Health Outreach; 2005.
51. Adelman HS, Taylor L. Mental health in schools and system restructuring. Clin Psychol Rev. 1999;19(2):137–63. doi:10.1016/S0272-7358(98)0007.
52. Elias MJ, Zins JE, Weissberg RP, Frey KS, Greenberg MT, Haynes NM, et al. Promoting social and emotional learning: guidelines for educators. Alexandria, VA: Association for Supervision and Curriculum Development; 1997.

53. Castro-Olivo SM, Merrell KW. Validating cultural adaptations of a school-based social-emotional learning programme for use with Latino immigrant adolescents. Adv Sch Ment Health Promot. 2012;5(2):78–92. doi:10.1080/1754730X.2012.6891.
54. Rousseau C, Drapeau A, Lacroix L, Bagilishya D, Heusch N. Evaluation of a classroom program of creative expression workshops for refugee and immigrant children. J Child Psychol Psychiatry. 2005;46(2):180–5. doi:10.1111/j.1469-7610.2004.00344.x.
55. Ellis BH, Miller AB, Abdi S, Barrett C, Blood EA, Betancourt TS. Multi-tier mental health program for refugee youth. J Consult Clin Psychol. 2012;81(1):129–40. doi:10.1037/a0029844.
56. Saxe GN, Ellis BH, Kaplow J. Collaborative care for traumatized teens and children: a trauma systems therapy approach. New York, NY: Guilford; 2006.
57. Acosta Price O, Ellis BH, Escudero PV, Huffman-Gottschling K, Sander MA, Birman D. Implementing trauma interventions in schools: addressing the immigrant and refugee experience. In: Notaro SR, editor. Health disparities among under-served populations: implications for research, policy and praxis (advances in education in diverse communities: research, policy and praxis, vol. 9. Bingley: Emerald Group Publishing; 2012. p. 95–119.
58. Stein BD, Kataoka SH, Jaycox LH, Wong M, Fink A, Escudero P, Zaragoza C. Theoretical basis and program design of a school-based mental health intervention for traumatized immigrant children: a collaborative research partnership. J Behav Health Serv Res. 2002;29(3):318–26. doi:10.1007/BF02287371.
59. Stein BD, Jaycox LH, Kataoka SH, Wong M, Tu W, Elliott MN, Fink A. A mental health intervention for school children exposed to violence: a randomized controlled trial. JAMA. 2003;290(5):603–11. doi:10.1001/jama.290.5.603.
60. Ringeisen H, Henderson K, Hoagwood K. Context matters: schools and the "research to practice gap" in children's mental health. Sch Psychol Rev. 2003;32(2):153–68.
61. Golden O, Fortuny K. Young children of immigrants and the path to educational success. Report on a roundtable. Washington, DC: The Urban Institute; 2011.
62. Ngo V, Langley A, Kataoka SH, Nadeem E, Escudero P, Stein BD. Providing evidence-based practice to ethnically diverse youths: examples from the cognitive behavioral intervention for trauma in schools (CBITS) program. J Am Acad Child Adolesc Psychiatry. 2008;47(8):858–62. doi:10.1097/CHI.0b013e3181799f19.

Trauma and Acculturative Stress

John P. Rettger, Hilit Kletter, and Victor Carrion

Abstract

There are a substantial number of immigrant youth living in the United States (USA), and there has been a recent media coverage documenting a rise in illegal entry by immigrants into the United States. Both legal and clandestine entries into the United States present various trauma risk factors for youth whose families seek the promise of a fruitful future in America. This chapter examines the various types of traumatic experiences immigrant youth may encounter, prevalent treatment approaches, and practical, community-based applications of treatment programs utilized by the Early Life Stress and Pediatric Anxiety Program at Stanford University. By investigating trauma before, during, and after migration, clinicians can achieve a greater depth of understanding on how to develop new treatment approaches and how to adapt existing psychotherapeutic models. Through an exploration of the psychosocial stressors immigrant youth face, various risk and resiliency factors during different phases of the migration process, potential comorbidities, and existing treatment models, we arrive at specific treatments and cultural adaptation recommendations.

Keywords

Immigrant youth • Trauma • Acculturative stress • Migrant youth • Refugee youth • Immigrant youth trauma treatment • Community-based mental health

J.P. Rettger, Ph.D. (✉) • H. Kletter, Ph.D. • V. Carrion, M.D.
Stanford Early Life Stress & Pediatric Anxiety Program, 401 Quarry Road, Room 3343,
Stanford, CA 94305-5719, USA
e-mail: jrettger@stanford.edu; hkletter@stanford.edu; vcarrion@stanford.edu

Introduction

The US Census Bureau [1] reports that approximately three million immigrant youth live in the United States. These youth are susceptible to a vast range of difficulties including identity crises, peer pressure, questions of self-worth, separation/loss, and parental conflict [2]. These difficulties place immigrant youth at a heightened risk for a variety of psychological problems including anxiety disorders, depression, substance use, conduct disorders, eating disorders, and post-traumatic stress disorder (PTSD) [3]. Immigrants can be roughly categorized into two groups: (1) those relocating by choice and having high socioeconomic status both in their country of origin and in the host country and (2) those forced to migrate and/or having low socioeconomic status in the country of origin. Both groups share similar difficulties such as adapting to a new language and culture; however, the second group is more vulnerable to trauma during all stages of the migration process.

Psychosocial Stress and Trauma

In this chapter, the discussion primarily focuses on trauma, which is distinct from psychosocial stressors. As defined and described previously in this book [4], immigrant youth life stressors include frequent [5] environmental events or conditions [6] that threaten physical, cognitive, and psychological health [7] and may exacerbate existing vulnerabilities related to previous trauma exposure [8]. Although stressors may not constitute a trauma, having multiple stressors accumulated across development may place the youth at a higher risk level for developing post-traumatic stress. This risk has been referred to as allostatic load [9].

For a diagnosis of PTSD, there must have been an identified trauma [10]. Psychological trauma may result from more extreme stressful events such as witnessing death or being threatened with a serious injury, sexual violence, or torture. These events may be witnessed, experienced directly, or occur through indirect exposure such as hearing about it through a friend, family member, or media coverage [11].

Symptoms of PTSD may include reexperiencing the event, avoidance of thoughts and feelings associated with the event, negative cognitions and mood, and increased reactivity. PTSD is especially of concern among immigrant youth since so many are exposed to witnessing or experiencing violence, physical or mental torture, death threats, extreme harassment, armed conflict, instability, hunger, and deprivation [12].

It is often assumed that youth adapt more easily to the immigration process [13]. However, immigrant youth are typically challenged by a bombardment of stressors that extend across intrapersonal, interpersonal, academic, social, and familial domains and are often experienced as a tension attempting to balance the extent to which they should preserve their original cultural identity and customs versus immersion in the new culture. They may feel pressured to blend in and to be more like their peers while discarding their own cultural customs and values [14]. Adopting the host country's attitudes and behaviors that are different from the ones expected in their native culture may lead to family conflict as youths' values clash with those of their parents [15].

It is important to keep in mind that stressors, acting across time, may constitute risk factors that contribute to development of post-traumatic stress symptoms. The complex relationships between psychosocial stressors and post-traumatic stress may impact what intervention may be most appropriate for a given population at a particular time. Therefore, the clinician must make careful consideration of these relationships during the assessment and intervention phase of treatment. There are also significant stressors and trauma that the youth may have been exposed to during the various stages of migration.

Stages of Migration and Trauma Risk

There are four stages of the migration process during which there is potential for trauma: (1) premigration (events immediately prior to migration that were the main determinant of relocation), (2) migration, (3) asylum seeking and resettlement, and (4) substandard living conditions in the new country due to unemployment, inadequate support, or persecution [16].

Premigration Risk Factors Researchers have reported on various psychosocial factors that may have been present for youth prior to migrating and that may have served as risk factors for the development of PTSD or other mental health symptoms. For instance, in a sample of US immigrant Latino adolescents and their primary caregivers, researchers have identified premigration poverty co-occurring with clandestine entry into the United States as risk factors for trauma and related PTSD symptom development [25]. Refugee youth are often exposed to severe trauma prior to migration such as violence exposure, food and water deprivation, family separation, and war atrocities [17]. During this phase, youth may experience the death of a family member or close relative, which may also increase the risk for developing trauma symptoms. The evidence suggests that the atrocities and dangers war-exposed [18–20] and refugee youth [21–23] are exposed to in their unstable home countries place them at risk for disorders or symptoms of PTSD, depression, anxiety, somatic complaints, sleep problems, and behavioral problems. Statistics suggest that these symptoms are more severe among youth with a higher level of exposure. Trauma research also informs us that those with a prior history of trauma are more vulnerable to the development of PTSD following an experience of a new trauma [24].

When considering the adversity experienced by premigratory youth, it may be surprising that evidence does exist that certain youth do not develop lasting adverse psychological effects. Researchers have identified several protective strategies that may be utilized to reduce trauma risks prior to migration. However, these factors are limited in application in that they describe the experiences of non-refugee youth. The potential risk of trauma exposure for youth may be reduced by parents adopting a migration strategy in which they leave their children with extended family in their home country until they can establish safe and/or legal means of migrating the youth [25]. In this scenario, parents may take sufficient time to adjust in the United States and to establish more financial stability. This strategy may reduce the risk of traumatic exposure; however, it does not necessarily stave off symptoms stemming from family separation, anxiety, and/or depression. Other protective factors that have been reported also include age (which is a complex variable that depends on numerous contextual factors, such as age at trauma exposure or age at migration and arrival into the resettlement country), familism, and higher levels of acculturation [25].

Migration Risks and Exposures Several hurdles arise during the migration process that may serve as risk factors for psychological stress. In a study by Perreira and Ornelas [26], they discovered that 29 % of foreign-born adolescents and 34 % of foreign-born parents experienced trauma during the migration process [25]. In a smaller subset of this sample, 9 % of adolescents and 21 % of their parents were reportedly at risk for PTSD.

Hardships endured during migration include traveling alone or with a smuggler, robbery, physical assault, illness, and accidental injury [26]. An increasing number of immigrants are promised paid passage, legal documentation, work, and housing by individuals either from their country of origin or host country who instead exploit them in the form of slavery, labor, or sex to make them pay off debt for these promises [2]. While many immigrants enter the host country legally, some have limited access to legal avenues due to poverty in their home countries and may have to enter without authorization [27]. Refugee youth who escape their home countries due to political, ethnic, and/or religious conflict especially lack the security of legality [2]. If unaccompanied, they often have to wait long periods in detention centers and may not be granted asylum (see chapter "Immigrant Youth and Navigating Unique Systems that Interact with Treatment" on social systems for more information), resulting in being sent back to the conditions of war, poverty, political massacres, and persecution in their homeland. Eighty to ninety percent of refugee youth witness murder or mass killings, endure forced labor, and are deprived of food for extreme periods of time [28]. In addition, they may experience combat, torture, forced separation from family, and life in refugee camps. Many immigrants endure long journeys with extreme physical hardship and exposure to violence [29].

Post-migration Upon integration into the new culture, there may be challenges associated with language, the social environment, and the separation from family and friends who they had to leave behind in their homeland [30]. Once youth have migrated and are beginning the process of acculturation, various stressors, such as the experience of discrimination, community violence, and unresolved psychological symptoms, must be coped with. For instance, in a study of 97 refugee youth in Australia, aged 11–19, researchers discovered that factors of belonging (in the Australian community), perceived discrimination, and bullying were of particular importance for subjective health and well-being outcomes for the refugees' first 3 years [31].

The role of discrimination in daily hardship is exemplified in Arab Muslim adolescents in immigrant families living in Euro-American countries [32]. Specifically, this group receives unfavorable media portrayal of their culture and religion. They report discrimination from peers and society and from the tension between Islamic and Euro-American norms about expected adolescent behavior [32–34].

Lastly, post-migration, families may end up living in unsafe neighborhoods. For example, in a study of 281 foreign-born adolescents and their parents residing in the

United States, post-migration discrimination and neighborhood disorder increased the risk of trauma exposure and the related emergence of PTSD symptoms [26].

The above research suggests that immigrant youth continue to face incredible challenges post-migration not only on a psychological level but also within their family, schools, and peer groups and also in their neighborhoods and community. Furthermore, post-migration, immigrant youth may struggle with learning a new language, shifts in roles and responsibilities, legal status, racism, and discrimination [26]. They may be segregated in impoverished and high-crime neighborhoods and schools where additional violence and discrimination occur [35].

Importance of Identifying Trauma and Related Comorbidity

The psychological issues presented by immigrant youth may be significant and compounded by exposure or, in some examples, by repetitive or chronic exposure to a range of traumatic experience. These youth may have survived war, torture, rape, physical and/or sexual abuse, and community violence before, during, and after migration. Such complex trauma exposure among these youth may contribute to higher rates of comorbidity. For example, Betancourt and colleagues [36] reported that in a youth sample from the National Child Traumatic Stress Network (NCTSN) Core Data Set of 60 war-affected refugee teenagers seeking psychological treatment, there were high rates of probable post-traumatic stress disorder (30.4 %), generalized anxiety (26.8 %), somatization (26.8 %), traumatic grief (21.4 %), and general behavioral problems (21.4 %). They also reported that those who were exposed to war or political violence were likely to have also experienced forced displacement, traumatic loss, bereavement or separation, exposure to community violence, and domestic violence. Academic problems (53.6 %) and behavioral difficulties (44.6 %) were also reported among these youth. Despite these adversities, criminal activity, alcohol/drug use, and self-harm were reported in less than 5.45 % of the sample.

The severity of traumatic exposure experienced by immigrant youth, the poor long-term prognosis of untreated post-traumatic stress, and the high-risk for comorbidity demand effective, culturally sensitive, and accessible treatment protocols. These protocols must take into account challenges such as assessment, valid and reliable diagnoses, and ethical issues of consent. Ideally, treatment interventions are designed for implementation at the levels of the community, family, school, and social support networks. Fortunately, there are numerous existing trauma treatment protocols that have been adapted by clinical researchers for immigrant youth.

Treatment Protocols for Immigrant Youth

The following section describes the prevalent trauma treatment interventions reported in the literature. Table 1, presented below, integrates key components that are utilized across interventions. The table has two sections. In the first section, general trauma treatment components are presented. In the second section, cultural

Table 1 Trauma treatment components

Treatment component	Description
Assessment and identification of youth in need of treatment [37]	• Culturally sensitive screening needs to occur early following a traumatic event • If possible, the use of multiple raters to examine subjective and objective perspectives while maintaining cultural sensitivity
Developing an understanding of the youth's cultural context [37]	• This understanding would include important relationships, community connections, spiritual and religious systems, as well as developmental and psychological history [38]
Psychoeducation components [39–42]	• Provide education to youth and caregivers on trauma and common reactions • Explain the treatment components and treatment plan • In appropriate language, explain the rationale for the skills learned in therapy and other treatment components • Provide the potential benefits of treatment
Relaxation and physiological training [39–42]	Instruction in basic relaxation skills, a few examples include: • Breathwork • Guided imagery • Mindfulness • Progressive muscle relaxation
Affect expression, regulation, and coping skills training; cognitive restructuring and processing [39–42]	Assist the youth in learning the process of: • Identifying and discerning specific emotions • Learn the distinction between thoughts and emotions • Instruct them on the role of thoughts, emotions, and physiological and behavioral reactions to situations or trauma reminders and how to cope with the full range of emotions • Teach skills in the communication of emotions and other internal states • Skills of empathy • Problem-solving skills training • Identify negative thoughts and cognitive distortion patterns and replace them with more positive and realistic thoughts
Behavioral change strategies [39, 40, 43]	• Instructing the youth on new, healthy, and more effective behavioral responses to trauma reminders
Trauma narrative [39, 40, 44]	• Facilitate the construction of a trauma narrative detailing the events of the trauma • Can utilize narration, writing, poetry, coloring, acting, song, or other preferred format • With youth's permission, the narrative is shared with the caregiver in the parallel session (if applicable)

(continued)

Table 1 (continued)

Treatment component	Description
Exposure work (imaginal, in vivo, or interoceptive) [39, 40, 44]	• Designing specific and appropriate gradual exposure strategies to eventually dissolve avoidance strategies of trauma reminders • Imaginal exposure involves the utilization of mental imagery • In vivo exposure utilizes a live, in-the-world strategy of confronting a trauma cue • Interoceptive exposure is the evoking of the physiological state triggered by a trauma cue and then practicing distress tolerance and relaxation training to cope with the physiological arousal
Caregiver-youth conjoint sessions and/or systems work [39, 40, 42, 43]	• Designed to strengthen the caregiver-youth relationship and develop more positive communication
Future planning and safety training [39, 40]	• Education and training designed to help the youth practice safety, healthy behaviors and decision-making, and danger assessment to avoid re-traumatization and re-victimization
Cultural adaptations of trauma components — see de Arellano et al. [45]	
Culturally specific systems engagement	• Increase the youth's, families', and communities' involvement through culturally sensitive treatment engagement strategies, as well as that of the community in a culturally sensitive way
Ongoing cultural sensitivity and rapport building in delivering treatment	• Establish a strong treatment alliance with participants through cultural awareness and relevant inclusion of cultural factors
Examining symptom expression through a cultural lens	• As part of treatment modules, such as psychoeducation, the clinician can educate the treatment participants on the common trauma reactions while making inclusion and consideration of how cultural factors may be influencing symptom expression
Appropriate and skillful use of interpreters, where indicated	• When essential treatment participants do not speak the same language as the therapist, it is critical to make appropriate use of translation services in order to effectively deliver treatment components with cultural sensitivity
Understanding cultural differences in emotional expression	• Cultural differences in emotional expression may include variations in the level of emotional expression and to whom it is considered appropriate to express the affect to • Clinicians may need to educate treatment participants on how to identify, regulate, and master emotional expression in a way that matches cultural expectations where appropriate

(continued)

Table 1 (continued)

Treatment component	Description
Culturally informed assessment of cultural views and relationship with cognitive processing or reframing	• The clinician needs to achieve an understanding of how cultural views may be acting to shape the youth's self-attributions or other related attributions following a traumatic event • Self-blame, guilt, and the belief that a caretaker failed in protecting them are examples of self-attributions or other attributions that may need processing
Culturally congruent construction of a coherent trauma narrative	• The clinician needs to evaluate what is the culturally appropriate communication of the trauma narrative to other family and community members to which the youth consents and wishes the narrative to be shared with
Drawing upon cultural supports for future planning, risk reduction, strength, and resiliency during the termination phase of treatment	• The clinician works to discover, utilize, and build upon the youth's, the family's, and community's existing strengths not only during treatment but also for ongoing healing after treatment termination • Treatment termination is characterized by the instilment of hope, optimism, empowerment, a sense of satisfaction, healthy closure, and preparedness for the future

adaptations are described. In practice, the implementation of trauma interventions can be complex with very specific, individual case differences. Therefore, the following table is a general guide and may not capture the full range of component combinations within a given treatment model. It can be used as a guide toward developing models or assessing current treatment paradigms for inclusion of critical components and cultural adaptations.

The above section provided a sweeping view of more universally present treatment components across trauma interventions. The following section includes concise summaries of a few of the more prevalent treatment protocols discussed in the literature. Those interested readers wishing to learn more in-depth information about these protocols can refer to the comprehensive review by de Arellano and colleagues [46] or the reference list to learn more about these approaches. A summary of these approaches is included in Table 2.

Parenting Through Change (PTC) PTC is an evidence-based intervention originally developed to prevent emotional and behavioral problems in children of separating parents [43]. It has been adapted for Latino and Somali parents affected by traumatic events [12, 47]. The 14-week parent management training emphasizes skills such as problem-solving, teaching through encouragement, limit setting, positive involvement, and child monitoring. PTC employs an active learning model in which group members role-play and practice strategies to acquire parenting skills. In addition to weekly group sessions, parents receive midweek calls from group facilitators to provide support and coaching. Cultural adaptations to PTC include

Table 2 Trauma interventions adapted for immigrant youth

Treatment	Immigrant groups	Cultural adaptations
Cognitive Behavioral Intervention for Trauma in Schools (CBITS)	• Latino (Mexico and Central America) • Korean • Russian • Western Armenian	• Language needs • Culturally relevant examples • Acceptance of differing beliefs • Spirituality • Sensitivity to migration trauma and acculturative stress • Increased family involvement • Cultural liaisons
Parenting Through Change (PTC)	• Latino • Somali	• Bilingual/bicultural providers • Teaching of skills to aid in acculturation • Narrative approach and storytelling • Cultural liaisons
Cultural Adjustment and Trauma Services (CATS)	• First- and second-generation immigrants from 29 countries	• Bicultural and/or bilingual providers • Cultural liaisons to provide outreach and case management • Address immigration, acculturation, and resettlement traumas
Culturally Modified Trauma-Focused Treatment (CM-TFT)	• Latino (Mexican, Central and South American)	• Wider range of traumas • Assess immigration, migration, and acculturation • Language needs • Family focus including extended family members • Address racism and discrimination • Gender roles • Spirituality • Folk beliefs and beliefs about mental health • Interpersonal style
Trauma Systems Therapy (TST)	• Latino (Mexico, Guatemala, Honduras) • Cambodian • Somali • Nigerian • Liberian • Sierra Leone • Ugandan	• Case management to build trust with providers • Language needs • Cultural liaisons • Cultural explanatory models of healing • Engagement through identification of cultural strengths

(1) placing bilingual/bicultural mental health professionals in schools to offer services, (2) working with community advocates and religious leaders to build trust with families and solicit feedback about helpful interventions, (3) using narrative approaches and storytelling to help youth and families process life events, and (4) conducting group activities to teach life skills such as acculturation. PTC has been found to improve parental emotion regulation, parenting practices, and parent interactions with their children [12]. In addition, youth had reduced disruptive school behaviors, fewer suspensions and office referrals, and increased school attendance and performance.

Trauma-Focused Cognitive Behavioral Therapy (TF-CBT) TF-CBT is among the most widely researched and used intervention for PTSD symptoms in youth and has been administered in individual, family, and group settings [48]. TF-CBT has been used in a comprehensive school-based mental health program [Cultural Adjustment and Trauma Services (CATS)] for first- and second-generation immigrant youth, and it was found to improve trauma symptoms and overall functioning [49]. Researchers modified TF-CBT for use with Latino immigrants (Culturally Modified Trauma-Focused Treatment, CM-TFT) [50]. According to the National Child Traumatic Stress Network (NCTSN) sources, the TF-CBT manual is being translated into Dutch and German and is being modified for children of Native American descent and for youth from other countries such as Zambia, Pakistan, the Netherlands, and Germany, among others [51]. Several of the measures used in TF-CBT have Spanish language translations. Adaptations made in CM-TFT include incorporating a wider range of traumas, an assessment of immigration and migration history, preferred language, acculturation for all family members, beliefs about mental health and treatment, and inclusion of all those involved in the care of the child in treatment. In addition, CM-TFT weaves in cultural constructs such as gender roles, spirituality, folk beliefs, interpersonal style, and family focus into treatment. A study of 32 Latino immigrant youth ages 7–17 with a history of sexual abuse, exposure to domestic violence, or traumatic grief found that CM-TFT was effective in reducing PTSD symptoms [50]. For more information on CBT applications for immigrant youth, please refer to "Chapter 2: Cognitive-Behavioral Therapy for Immigrant Youth: The Essentials" of this text.

Trauma Systems Therapy (TST) TST is a comprehensive treatment approach that assesses and treats child trauma by focusing on social and environmental factors that are thought to be impacting the child's emotional and behavioral functioning [52]. The social context, including the family, school, and neighborhood, are the components of the *trauma system*. Children as young as 3 years old have been treated with TST, and treatment ranges in length for up to 11 months. Several studies have examined the effects of TST. In a 2004 open trial study of 110 urban and rural youth aged between 5 and 20, researchers found significant improvements on clinician ratings of children's psychiatric symptoms and their social environment after 3 months of TST [42]. Another study compared TST to care as usual (CAU) in retaining a group of urban youth ($n = 20$) treatment participants with elevated post-traumatic stress symptoms. The researchers found that after the 3-month assessment, 90 % of the TST participants were retained, a far superior percentage to the 10 % of CAU participants retained [53]. This finding is noteworthy considering that up to 90 % of traumatized youth living in urban settings may terminate treatment early [54]. Project SHIFA (Supporting the Health of Immigrant Families and Adolescents) utilized the TST model to provide secondary prevention and intervention services to Somali immigrant youth, resulting in a significant reduction in trauma symptoms and improvement in emotional regulation [55]. A specific adaptation of TST exists for refugees and immigrants called TST-R [56]. In this application, TST services are delivered at an appropriate level of care, such as school or home based, with the use of either cultural providers from the same community as the youth or cultural brokers, who may be paraprofessionals paired with a clinician who may not be a member of the youth's community.

Table 2 presents the immigrant groups and cultural adaptations for which the above treatment interventions have been adapted.

Examining the range of cultural adaptations for existing trauma treatment protocols through the lens of the migration experience illuminates several factors toward which treatment recommendations can be made. The next section highlights important considerations that clinicians are encouraged to include while determining their treatment plan.

Treatment Recommendations

According to the Workgroup on Adapting Latino Services [57] report, when treating immigrant youth, it is especially important to assess all experiences throughout the migration process. To that end, Delgado and colleagues [58] proposed eight factors that need to be considered in treatment planning and intervention development for immigrant youth: (1) original culture, (2) country of origin, (3) premigration life, (4) circumstances of migration, (5) trauma experience, (6) family fragmentation, (7) legal status and resettlement process, and (8) host community. Aside from evaluating stressors related to the migration process, clinicians should also assess issues related to basic needs, family functioning, trauma symptoms, immigration, and documentation status. For instance, clinicians provide resources and referrals to services that can assist with housing and shelter, food, clothing, childcare, and education. Research evidence makes clear the need for integrated services, specialized treatment centers for immigrants, and a multidisciplinary team providing care that can address the range of treatment needs. Differences in adaptation between immigrant youth and their parents should also be assessed as youth often adjust to the host country more quickly than their parents, which may lead to conflict. Certainly as part of treatment planning, the clinician must also be aware of specific cultural considerations that may bear influence on the therapy relationship and treatment outcomes. Several of these considerations are noted in the following section.

Cultural Considerations   Trauma clinicians need to familiarize themselves with the cultural values of the immigrant community as these provide the basis for understanding the attitudes, beliefs, and decisions of youth and their families [2]. This may include assessing attitudes about mental health and treatment as well as spirituality, folk beliefs, family focus, and gender roles [59]. In addition, language needs should be addressed and may include using bilingual/bicultural clinicians or interpreters, reducing the need for written language through storytelling or narrative approaches, and using visual aids. Furthermore, clinicians need to consider differing cultural beliefs and need to not discount those beliefs if appropriate to the youth's culture.

Treatment content should not conflict with the cultural values of the immigrant community and ought to provide culturally relevant examples [12]. Using a cultural broker who has clinical experience and familiarity with the immigrant community may help to build trust, provide a guide to immigrant traditions and beliefs, and bridge communication. Furthermore, establishing community partnerships and focus groups comprised of individuals from the immigrant culture may help inform: (1) existing engagement strategies (2) address specific cultural issues, (3) guide understanding on how to introduce treatment, and (4) identify potential barriers to intervention [41].

Thus far, this chapter has discussed a number of existing treatments and cultural adaptations; in the following section, specific examples of how these concepts are being applied in the community-based intervention work at the Stanford University School of Medicine's Early Life Stress and Pediatric Anxiety Program (ELSPAP). As part of daily operations, the ELSPAP team interacts with immigrant youth and families in each program, and several strategies are utilized to build and maintain strong community partnerships through which culturally sensitive adaptations for treatment approaches were developed.

Stanford Early Life Stress and Pediatric Anxiety Program

The ELSPAP engages in numerous projects serving immigrant families and youth. The interventions developed were not specifically designed for immigrant youth populations per se; however, through clinical practice and direct service delivery, effective adaptations were developed. The populations served include the Ravenswood City School District (RCSD) in East Palo Alto (EPA), California, charter schools, and nonprofit agencies. In addition to the EPA community, ELSPAP engages in ongoing consulting and staff support services at the Center for Youth Wellness (CYW) in San Francisco, CA, and has other national and international collaborators. The CYW is a trauma-informed mental health treatment center serving youth survivors of traumatic experience and their families in the Bayview community of San Francisco. Two of these unique programs, the Stanford Cue-Centered Treatment and the ELSPAP Mindfulness program, and their implementation models are described below.

Stanford Cue-Centered Treatment (CCT) CCT is a manualized protocol designed for youth ages 8–18, who have experienced repeated exposure to traumatic events [39]. It consists of 15–18 weekly individual sessions, designed to last approximately 50 min in duration. CCT is an integrative approach, combining elements from cognitive, behavioral, psychodynamic, expressive, and family therapies to address four core domains (cognition, behavior, emotions, and physiology). The primary goal of CCT is to build strength and resilience by empowering the youth through knowledge regarding the relationship between their history of trauma exposure and current affective, cognitive, behavioral, or physiological responses. In CCT, the youth is asked to create a life timeline to help the youth examine the impact of multiple traumas and daily life stressors. In addition, CCT teaches the youth to become aware of their interoceptive cues that include heart rate and breathing in order to help them better identify their emotions.

A recent randomized controlled study in 13 high-risk, low-income schools in San Francisco and East Palo Alto examined the efficacy of CCT as a short-term intervention for youth with a history of chronic interpersonal violence [39]. Results from the study showed decreased post-traumatic stress (both youth and parent reported), anxiety, and depression symptoms, as well as an overall improvement of functioning as rated by the therapists, while caregivers had differential reductions in anxiety and depression.

A number of adaptations have been made to CCT for use with immigrant youth, primarily Latino of Mexican or Central American origin. The treatment manual, handouts, and assessments have all been translated into Spanish. While administering the translated assessments, many caregivers informed the researchers that they understood what the questions were asking yet it would be worded differently in Spanish. Thus, it is important to ensure that culturally appropriate terms are used. Visual aids are also helpful in overcoming language barriers. For example, CCT uses a picture thermometer to have youth rate feelings and worksheets use visual depictions to explain concepts such as the cognitive square (i.e., four core domains of trauma). Cultural brokers with mental health experience and knowledge of the immigrant community were identified at each school to serve as liaisons to help initiate contact with families, understand their needs, and translate during treatment sessions. Successful treatment also included community engagement such as involvement of community leaders, attendance at back-to-school nights and parent meetings to build a relationship with the families, and psychoeducational workshops for school staff on recognizing trauma in immigrant youth and how to mitigate its effects.

Treatment incorporated the youth's own cultural beliefs and values and included culturally relevant examples. For instance, many of the youth are active in church groups and strongly believe in the power of prayer; thus, prayer was added to their coping toolkit. Another example is that for many of the youth, traditional foods hold significant meaning and are associated with a sense of family. To be respectful of this custom, clinicians invited families to share these foods in the treatment sessions, which often broke the ice and made families feel more at home. Finally, trauma symptoms may be manifested in a variety of ways depending on the culture; therefore, a youth's experience should not be dismissed no matter how different or odd it may appear. An example of this is that it is not uncommon for Latino youth to believe in visions or ghosts, and if a clinician were to simply treat this as another symptom, it might lead to the assessment of the youth for a psychotic disorder. Therefore, symptoms must be taken in the context of the culture.

Case Study

The following case illustrates an application of the CCT psychotherapy model for an immigrant youth and his mother. Certain insignificant details of the case have been modified to protect confidentiality. Francisco is a 14-year-old male of Columbian origin who witnessed his father beating his mother while the father was under the influence of drugs and alcohol while living in their home in Columbia. At the time of the incident, Francisco was 5 years old.

The CCT intervention was being delivered to Francisco at his school. Typically, ELSPAP research staff utilizes cultural mediators at the schools to make initial contacts with or to inform the families about our program. Using familiar community members as cultural mediators facilitates trust between the family and program staff. Spanish-speaking research staff are utilized to provide translation services for clinicians. It is also common for researchers and clinicians to have close relationships with school personnel, particularly the school office managers. This type of relationship promotes more effective communication with families, since the office managers tend to interact with and see the families frequently at school. Many of the parents of the youth in ELSPAP programs are Spanish speaking. Therefore, utilizing the school staff, who are Spanish-speaking community members and who at often times are willing to act as translators, helps to facilitate rapport with families upon initial contact.

During the initial assessment and intake, the parent reported that Francisco was doing well prior to the trauma. During episodes of violence between his father and mother, Francisco would retreat to his bedroom and would not come back out from his room. This was also how Francisco behaved when his father was under the influence of alcohol. Subsequent to the trauma, the mother reported that Francisco began to get into frequent trouble at school for fighting and tagging (graffiti). The mother reported that on numerous occasions, the father threatened to take the children away from her. The family reported strong social supports of family members and friends, but no community-based support. This kind of data gathering that occurs during the CCT assessment phase provides an opportunity to learn about the particular cultural values and resources of the family. In this case, there is strong family support but a lack of community support. Therefore, the therapist can work to understand how to utilize family supports and work in collaboration with the family to develop a support system in their community. The assessment phase is also a doorway to discuss how the family's cultural background may influence the expression of affect, affection, communication, and the key family members who may act as treatment allies.

According to the mother, she had become more sad and nervous following being physically abused by the father. The clinician experienced difficulty in conducting the assessment due to language barriers with the mother. To overcome this language barrier between the clinician and Francisco's mother, the clinician worked to have an interpreter available as a best practice. However in this particular case, there was not an appropriate interpreter at the school, and therefore, Francisco acted as a translator for the mother. The therapist noted that this additional level of involvement seemed to spark an attentiveness and curiosity about the treatment protocol. In this case, the use of the youth as a translator seemed to have a positive effect. A potential limitation of this strategy is that it may place the youth in more of an adult role as well as exposing the youth to additional emotional stress. This evidence of rapport and engagement with the mother is apparent in her asking for substance abuse treatment referrals for her oldest son, whom she feared was using. Providing referrals is another opportunity in which the CCT protocol can include culturally relevant materials and connections to appropriate community resources. At the end of the assessment, psychoeducation materials were provided to the mother in Spanish.

By the completion of the second session, Francisco had placed 11 tools in his toolbox, including the common core of CCT tools taught to youth such as progressive muscle relaxation and deep breathing and self-generated tools of talking with siblings, spending time with his mom, playing football or soccer, and writing. The CCT toolbox provides an excellent opportunity for the clinician to include cultural adaptations. For instance, the clinician may ask the youth about culturally specific resources that may be included such as church community, religious or spiritual sources of strength, prayer, traditional music, and activities. Francisco used deep breathing to help soothe himself during conflicts with siblings; he imagined using positive thoughts to work his way through difficult homework assignments as well as being able to generate positive thoughts to replace negative ones.

By the conclusion of treatment, Francisco was able to talk about witnessing his mother being beaten by his father without the various cognitive distortions present in his first narrative. Positive effects of treatment were also noticeable in Francisco's *body map of feelings*. The body map is an outline of a human figure in which specific emotions are given a color and mapped onto the body. In particular, Francisco's map had a much greater surface area of love and happiness and somewhat of a smaller surface area of challenging emotions such as anger and worry when compared to baseline. The conclusion of treatment provides an additional opportunity to connect the family with cultural resources that may provide protective factors against future stressors.

Stanford Mindfulness Program The mindfulness program was developed to provide additional mental health support in the Ravenswood City School District (RCSD). The RCSD is a predominately Latino (79 %) district with approximately 3500 kindergarten through eighth grade students and a child development center. Historically, the East Palo Alto community has suffered from extensive gang violence and poverty. The following quote poignantly describes concerns in the EPA community; the text was painted on the side of one of the district school buildings:

"Kids now a days want to be what they see on T.V. Remember there is more to life than looking cool. Many people in this world face things you don't even think about like my friends' boy's mom took her own life, the amount of children committing suicide because of bullying, kids parents on drugs, sexual abuse, kids starving. If you want to be different than the usual, make a difference and be nice. Today try not to think about yourself, but think about how you can help. You have no idea how you could make someone's day. I know there is a lot of violence in East Palo Alto, but this community has a lot of potential. Make your difference to the world, and your world will make a difference for you."

This statement specifically names many of the devastating issues discussed in this chapter and also perhaps more importantly points to the hope felt in the community that healing and positive transformation are possible. It calls upon not only the effort of the individual in creating change, but also it evokes community spirit in pulling together to create change. It is that sense of hope, resiliency, and optimism that our mindfulness program aims to cultivate in the youth.

Therefore, the specific goals of the youth and adult mindfulness programs are to (1) increase participants' self-awareness and self-regulation; (2) teach the mindfulness student to understand the interconnectedness of thoughts, emotions, physical sensations, and behaviors and how stress impacts functioning in these areas; (3) instruct mindfulness-based practices; (4) cultivate empathy and compassion; and (5) teach effective coping tools, such as relaxation skills, yoga, self-compassion and other compassion practices, and breathwork.

The pilot program reached 213 third and fourth graders across nine classrooms, with each classroom receiving 30 min of mindfulness instruction once per week over an 8-week period in the general school classroom. Pilot research results demonstrated statistically significant improvements for students reporting baseline risk or clinically significant scores on internalizing problems, inattention/hyperactivity, emotional symptoms, and personal adjustment. A number of these functional areas also were related to significant improvements in other areas for those who exhibited elevated risk at baseline. Examples from student journal reflections included: "What I learned was when I'm mad I can feel calm and be happy" and "If I got mad I breathe in and out to calm me down." Student journal entries reflect the positive influence of the program on their emotions and also suggest that younger children understand how to employ mindfulness practices outside of the school setting. One student wrote about how she taught yoga poses to her cousin. The full study findings will be published in a forthcoming article. Study limitations included a simple, correlational pre-post design without a control group, however, positive student feedback, and the mostly enthusiastic reception of the program by district staff suggests the program was successful.

Due to the extensive nature of the ELSPAP research efforts, assessment process, and interventions, it is critical that the community members and research participants receive culturally appropriate and comprehendible information about the programs and research goals. To support this effort, the program staff includes several Spanish-speaking members. As part of recruitment and ongoing operations, relationships are continuously being developed with the community members, school staff, and parents.

Conclusion

Immigrant youth typically face numerous traumatic stressors and experiences before, during, and after their migratory journey to the United States or other resettlement countries. Researchers and clinicians working with this population must be able to make careful and culturally sensitive assessments and treatment planning decisions that recognize and honor the traditions and experiences of the youth and their families. By examining existing research evidence, we are able to appreciate the complexity of traumatic experience, comorbidities, and existing treatments; we can gain insight into how to best approach intervention at the individual, family, and community levels. Forming strong relationships with community members and organizations and approaching assessment and treatment with openness and curiosity about the cultural traditions and acculturative experiences of youth and their families enable the mental health professional to be aware of the challenges that may serve as treatment barriers. Subsequently, we can design sustainable interventions and programs that may be used to sensitively work through access obstacles and successfully engage the youth, families, and community members to create healthier communities.

References

1. Bureau UC. Selected characteristics of the native and foreign born populations, S0501. Washington, DC: US Census Bureau; 2010.
2. Fong R. Immigrant and refugee youth: migration journeys and cultural values. The Prev Res. 2007;14(4):3–5.
3. Pumariega AJ, Rothe E, Pumariega JB. Mental health of immigrants and refugees. Community Ment Health J. 2005;41(5):581–97.
4. Staudenmeyer A, Macciomei E, del Cid M, Patel SG. Immigrant youth life stressors. In: Patel S, Reicherter D, editors. Psychotherapy for Immigrant Youth. New York, NY: Springer; 2015.
5. Pratt L, Barling J. Differentiating between daily events, acute and chronic stressors: a framework and its implications. In: Hurrell Jr JJ, Murphy LR, Sauter SL, Cooper CL, editors. Occupational stress: issues and developments in research. London: Taylor & Francis; 1988. p. 41–53.
6. Grant KE, Compas BE, Stuhlmacher AF, Thurm AE, McMahon SD, Halpert JA. Stressors and child and adolescent psychopathology: moving from markers to mechanisms of risk. Psychol Bull. 2003;129(3):447.
7. Sapolsky RM. Why zebras don't get ulcers: The acclaimed guide to stress, stress-related diseases, and coping-now revised and updated. Macmillan; 2004.
8. Kubiak SP. Trauma and cumulative adversity in women of a disadvantaged social location. Am J Orthopsychiatry. 2005;75(4):451.
9. McEwen BS. Allostasis and allostatic load: implications for neuropsychopharmacology. Neuropsychopharmacology. 2000;22(2):108–24.
10. Diagnostic and statistical manual of mental disorders. 5th Ed. American Psychiatric Association; 2013.
11. Schuster MA, Stein BD, Jaycox LH, Collins RL, Marshall GN, Elliott MN, et al. A national survey of stress reactions after the September 11, 2001, terrorist attacks. N Engl J Med. 2001;345(20):1507–12.
12. Gewirtz A, Mohammad J, Orieny P, Yaylaci F. Adapting trauma interventions for refugee families. The Dialogue. 2011;7:2–3.

13. Berry JW. Immigration, acculturation, and adaptation. Appl Psychol. 1997;46(1):5–34.
14. Igoa C. The inner world of the immigrant child. New York: St. Martin's Press; 1995.
15. Baptiste J, David A. Immigrant families, adolescents and acculturation: insights for therapists. Marriage Fam Rev. 1993;19(3-4):341–63.
16. Foster RP. When immigration is trauma: guidelines for the individual and family clinician. Am J Orthopsychiatry. 2001;71(2):153.
17. Measham T, Guzder J, Rousseau C, Pacione L, Blais-McPherson M, Nadeau L. Refugee children and their families: supporting psychological well-being and positive adaptation following migration. Curr Probl Pediatr Adolesc Health Care. 2014;44(7):208–15.
18. Jensen PS, Shaw J. Children as victims of war: current knowledge and future research needs. J Am Acad Child Adolesc Psychiatry. 1993;32(4):697–708.
19. Shaw JA. Children exposed to war/terrorism. Clin Child Fam Psychol Rev. 2003;6(4):237–46.
20. Stichick T. The psychosocial impact of armed conflict on children: rethinking traditional paradigms in research and intervention. Child Adolesc Psychiatr Clin N Am. 2001;10(4):797–814.
21. Athey JL, Ahearn FL. The mental health of refugee children: an overview. In: Ahearn FL, Athey JL, editors. Refugee children: theory, research and services. Baltimore: John Hopkins University Press; 1991. p. 3–19.
22. Keyes E. Mental health status in refugees: an integrative review of current research. Issues Ment Health Nurs. 2000;21:397–410.
23. Rousseau C. The mental health of refugee children. Transcult Psychiatry. 1995;32(3):299–331.
24. Breslau N, Chilcoat HD, Kessler RC, Davis GC. Previous exposure to trauma and PTSD effects of subsequent trauma: results from the Detroit Area Survey of Trauma. Am J Psychiatry. 2014;156(6):902–7.
25. Perreira KM, Ornelas IJ. Painful passages: traumatic experiences and post-traumatic stress among US Immigrant Latino adolescents and their primary caregivers. Int Migr Rev. 2013;47(4):976–1005.
26. Perreira KM, Ornelas IJ. The physical and psychological well-being of immigrant children. Futur Child. 2011;21(1):195–218.
27. Riosmena F, Massey DS. Pathways to El Norte: origins, destinations, and characteristics of Mexican Migrants to the United States. Int Migr Rev. 2012;46(1):3–36.
28. Lustig SL, Kia-Keating M, Knight WG, Geltman P, Ellis H, Kinzie JD, et al. Review of child and adolescent refugee mental health. J Am Acad Child Adolesc Psychiatry. 2004;43(1):24–36.
29. Infante C, Idrovo AJ, Sánchez-Domínguez MS, Vinhas S, González-Vázquez T. Violence committed against migrants in transit: experiences on the northern Mexican border. J Immigr Minor Health. 2012;14(3):449–59.
30. Gudiño OG, Nadeem E, Kataoka SH, Lau AS. Relative impact of violence exposure and immigrant stressors on Latino youth psychopathology. J Commun Psychol. 2011;39(3):316–35.
31. Correa-Velez I, Gifford SM, Barnett AG. Longing to belong: social inclusion and wellbeing among youth with refugee backgrounds in the first three years in Melbourne, Australia. Soc Sci Med. 2010;71(8):1399–408. doi:10.1016/j.socscimed.2010.07.018.
32. Aroian K, Templin T, Hough E. Longitudinal study of daily hassles in adolescents in Arab Muslim immigrant families. J Immigr Minor Health. 2014;16(5):831–8. doi:10.1007/s10903-013-9795-7.
33. Britto PR. Who am I? Ethnic identity formation of Arab Muslim children in contemporary US society. J Am Acad Child Adolesc Psychiatry. 2008;47(8):853–7.
34. Naber N. The rules of forced engagement race, gender, and the culture of fear among Arab immigrants in San Francisco post-9/11. Cult Dyn. 2006;18(3):235–67.
35. Oropesa R. Neighbourhood disorder and social cohesiveness among immigrants in a new destination Dominicans in Reading, PA. Urban Stud. 2012;49(1):115–32.
36. Betancourt TS, Newnham EA, Layne CM, Kim S, Steinberg AM, Ellis H, Birman D. Trauma history and psychopathology in war-affected refugee children referred for trauma-related mental health services in the United States. J Trauma Stress. 2012;25(6):682–90.
37. Kletter H, Rialon RA, Laor N, Brom D, Pat-Horenczyk R, Shaheen M, et al. Helping children exposed to war and violence: perspectives from an international work group on interventions for youth and families. Paper presented at the Child and Youth Care Forum; 2013.

38. Barenbaum J, Ruchkin V, Schwab-Stone M. The psychosocial aspects of children exposed to war: practice and policy initiatives. J Child Psychol Psychiatry. 2004;45(1):41–62.
39. Carrion VG, Kletter H, Weems CF, Berry RR, Rettger JP. Cue-centered treatment for youth exposed to interpersonal violence: a randomized controlled trial. J Trauma Stress. 2013;26(6):654–62.
40. Cohen JA, Mannarino AP. Trauma-focused cognitive behavioural therapy for children and parents. Child Adolesc Mental Health. 2008;13(4):158–62.
41. Ngo V, Langley A, Kataoka SH, Nadeem E, Escudero P, Stein BD. Providing evidence based practice to ethnically diverse youth: Examples from the Cognitive Behavioral Intervention for Trauma in Schools (CBITS) program. J Am Acad Child Adolesc Psychiatry. 2008;47(8):858.
42. Saxe GN, Ellis BH, Fogler J, Hansen S, Sorkin B. Comprehensive care for traumatized children-an open trial examines a specialized treatment plan--trauma systems therapy. Psychiatr Ann. 2005;35(5):443–9.
43. Forgatch MS, DeGarmo DS. Parenting through change: an effective prevention program for single mothers. J Consult Clin Psychol. 1999;67(5):711.
44. Neuner F, Catani C, Ruf M, Schauer E, Schauer M, Elbert T. Narrative exposure therapy for the treatment of traumatized children and adolescents (KidNET): from neurocognitive theory to field intervention. Child Adolesc Psychiatr Clin N Am. 2008;17(3):641–64.
45. de Arellano M, Ko S, Danielson C, Sprague C (2008). Trauma-informed interventions: clinical and research evidence and culture-specific information project. Retrieved from: http://www. nctsn.org/nctsn_assets/pdfs/CCG_Book.pdf
46. de Arellano M, Ko S, Danielson C, Sprague C (2008). Trauma-informed interventions: clinical and research evidence and culture-specific information project.
47. Gewirtz A, Taylor T. Participation of homeless and abused women in a parent training program: Science and practice converge in a battered women's shelter. In: Hindsworth MF, Lang TB, editors. Community participation and empowerment. Hauppage, NY: Nova Science; 2009. p. 97–114.
48. Cohen J, Deblinger E, Mannarino A, Steer R. A multi-site, randomized controlled trial for sexually abused children with PTSD symptoms. J Am Acad Child Adolesc Psychiatry. 2004;43:393–402.
49. Beehler S, Birman D, Campbell R. The effectiveness of cultural adjustment and trauma services (CATS): generating practice-based evidence on a comprehensive, school-based mental health intervention for immigrant youth. Am J Community Psychol. 2012;50(1–2):155–68.
50. Rivera S, de Arellano M. Culturally modified trauma-focused treatment for hispanic children: preliminary findings. Paper presented at the International Conference on Child and Family Maltreatment, San Diego, CA; 2008.
51. Trauma-Focused Cognitive Therapy (TF-CBT) (2007, 03/20/2007) from http://www.nctsn. org/nctsn_assets/pdfs/promising_practices/TF-CBT_fact_sheet_3-20-07.pdf
52. Brown A, Navalta, CP, Tullberg, E, & Saxe, G. Trauma systems therapy: an approach to creating trauma-informed child welfare systems. In: Reece RM, Hanson RF, Sargent J, editors. Treatment of child abuse: common ground for mental health, medical, and legal practitioners. Baltimore, MD: Johns Hopkins University Press; 2014. 132–138.
53. Saxe GN, Ellis BH, Fogler J, Navalta CP. Innovations in practice: preliminary evidence for effective family engagement in treatment for child traumatic stress–trauma systems therapy approach to preventing dropout. Child Adolesc Mental Health. 2012;17(1):58–61.
54. McKay MM, Lynn CJ, Bannon WM. Understanding inner city child mental health need and trauma exposure: implications for preparing urban service providers. Am J Orthopsychiatry. 2005;75(2):201.
55. Ellis BH, Miller AB, Baldwin H, Abdi S. New directions in refugee youth mental health services: overcoming barriers to engagement. J Child Adolesc Trauma. 2011;4(1):69–85.
56. Refugees and Immigrants. from https://www.med.nyu.edu/child-adolescent-psychiatry/research/ institutes-and-programs/trauma-and-resilience-research-program/trauma-systems-therapy-7
57. The Workgroup on Adapting Latino Services. Adaptation guidelines for serving Latino children and families affected by trauma. 1st ed. San Diego, CA: Chadwick Center for Children and Families; 2008.
58. Delgado M, Jones K, Rohani M. Social work practice with refugee and immigrant youth. Boston, MA: Allyn and Bacon Press; 2005.
59. Rivera S. Culturally-modified trauma-focused treatment for Hispanic children: Preliminary findings: ProQuest; 2007.

Part III

Interventions Complimentary to Psychotherapy for Immigrant Youth

Combined Psychotherapy with Psychopharmacology

Yasmin Owusu

Abstract

Medication prescribing in immigrant youth populations both reveals and engages very complex dynamics of family and culture. When pursuing psychopharmacologic intervention, the pharmacotherapist must be attuned to this array of elaborate dynamics. Understanding the significance of medication to the patient and their associated family system is incredibly informative to the conceptualization of the case. Psychological meanings will be embedded in many aspects of the pharmacotherapeutic process, and the prescribing clinician must remain curious about these meanings. This chapter will discuss how to examine context in the pharmacotherapeutic process, common dynamics to explore, issues around autonomy that arise, as well as collaborative care models of medication and psychotherapy treatment planning.

Keywords

Pharmacotherapy • Psychopharmacology • Medication • Explanatory models • Autonomy • Consent • Treatment alliance • Collaborative care

Pharmacotherapy: Essentials

There are many clinical circumstances in which consideration must be made for the addition of psychotropic agents to the comprehensive treatment plan of our child and adolescent patients. Psychiatric medications can be effective in relieving the suffering caused by distressing symptoms such as mood changes, anxiety,

Y. Owusu, M.D. (✉)
Department of Psychiatry, Stanford University, Stanford, CA, USA
e-mail: yowusu@stanford.edu

© Springer International Publishing Switzerland 2016
S.G. Patel, D. Reicherter (eds.), *Psychotherapy for Immigrant Youth*,
DOI 10.1007/978-3-319-24693-2_6

agitation, insomnia, psychosis, and other disturbances. It is essential that a comprehensive assessment be made by a qualified clinician to determine the appropriateness of a pharmacologic treatment approach. Such an assessment should be thorough and nuanced. This is the case for any psychiatric treatment scenario but becomes particularly true with special populations including children/adolescents and immigrant families [1]. With the identified patient being a minor, family dynamics and cultural context interact with the clinical process and imbue decisions with added complexity [2]. Pharmacologic clinical decision-making must be considered with care and diligent curiosity [3].

Respect Context The fundamental guiding principle in assessing the role of medication prescribing to the unique population of immigrant youth is to *respect context*. The context in which medications are prescribed has incredible psychological meaning to patients and their families [4]. This is the case in the sense of both developmental and social context. The meanings patients and families attribute to medications are important to the care. This importance cannot be underestimated. It is essential for prescribing clinicians to be attuned to these meanings [4]. It is crucial for all clinicians to have authentic interest in exploring this meaning. In any individual case, thoughtful consideration of the many contextual nuances and their associated psychological meanings should serve as the primary rudder for all clinical treatment decisions [5, 6].

Pharmacotherapy Prescribing clinicians should be deliberate in examining their identity and role in the treatment team as they embark on the care of immigrant youth populations. The prescribing provider can begin with an exploration of the nomenclature associated with his/her identity. *Do you identify yourself as a "prescriber"? A "pharmacologist"?* Consider the value in embracing an alternative term and thus a more broad-spectrum identity—*pharmacotherapist* [5]. There is incredible value and potential energy permeating such a title because it embraces a hybrid space. It orients the clinician to the previously stated guiding principles—respect context and understand the psychological meaning associated with any medication prescription.

As suggested by Gabbard and Kay [7], the *pharmacotherapist* must be "conceptually bilingual" in the language of both biology and psychology. The pharmacotherapist must embrace being much more than a prescriber. The pharmacotherapist is limber in her skill set and attuned to the biological needs of the patient and the interpersonal dynamics of the patient and family. With agility, the pharmacotherapist investigates both the biological sphere and the psychological sphere of any treatment context. Among the many unique potential cultural spaces that this patient population presents, this juncture between biology and psychology can very well be considered a cultural interface of its own.

Immigrant youth typically only come to the attention of a pharmacotherapist when a significant amount of distress has permeated the life of the identified patient and their family [1]. There can be a compulsion to quickly reach for a prescription pad with the hopes that it might be the cooling salve to a heated and anguished situation. The job of the pharmacotherapist is in part to do what can feel far from instinctive—slow down and gather more information. This is the time for the pharmacotherapist to actively explore the explanatory models of illness present in each case.

Explanatory Models An explanatory model explores how people make sense of their illness, including its cause. As defined by Arthur Kleinman, these models are "the beliefs the patient holds about his illness, the personal and social meaning he attaches to his disorder, his expectations about what will happen to him and what the doctor will do, and his own therapeutic goals" [8]. The key idea is that all involved parties in a single clinical scenario have an explanatory model, and they could all be distinctly different [9]. The patient, family members, and the physician will each have an explanatory model. At times, the explanatory models of various stakeholders will be in alignment. But not surprisingly, the explanatory models often may be divergent among stakeholders. The pharmacotherapist can work to identify where the discrepancies exist and then assist in negotiating these spaces.

For example, if a pharmacotherapist discovers in their inquiry that the family's explanatory model is not highly biologic, the pharmacotherapist should consider whether a medication prescription would be viewed by the family as having little value. The pharmacotherapist might find in such a case that if a prescription is written, it may not ever be filled by the family. Alternatively, if the pharmacotherapist sees the etiology of clinical symptoms as fundamentally sociocultural, the pharmacotherapist may steer clear of medication, even if it is desired by the patient or family.

Psychiatric Culture Returning to the guiding principle of respecting context, pharmacotherapists must act as ethnographers of the patient and family's cultural milieu, just as the patient and family might be likened to ethnographers of the psychiatric culture [3]. Especially in the case of immigrant youth, the potential for cultural differences is high [9]. Many will come from cultural backgrounds where medical models and psychiatric care in general are de-emphasized [10]. Pumariega in his Practice Parameters for Cultural Competence in Child and Adolescent Psychiatry [1] reminds us that, for example, families from Latino cultures may be apprehensive of psychiatric care because "perceptions of mental illness (including stigma and beliefs about causality), fatalism, spirituality, 'familism' (in which the family is considered the primary unit of identification and allegiance and leads to keeping problems within the family), cultural commitment (e.g., to using only culturally sanctioned helping approaches)" (p. 1103) all can seem to compete with the psychiatric medical model. It is wise to collaboratively explore with the family and patient what their hopes and fears are for the pharmacotherapy journey up ahead. It is this authentic engagement and curiosity that underlies the treatment alliance and in turn the foundation of the prescribing experience.

Formulation Pruett et al. [11] remind us that "the formulation should precede the prescription" (p. 431). Prescribing providers must put as much effort as possible into comprehensively conceptualizing the case before writing medication prescriptions. This includes a concerted effort to acknowledge culture as a foundation of that formulation. The prescriber will be better off over the course of treatment if they as a pharmacotherapist understand the symptoms as well as possible before actually treating them. However, one also must retain flexibility enough to refine that formulation over time and course correct as necessary.

The process of pharmacotherapy decision-making is often influenced by many stakeholders including the prescribing physician, child/adolescent patient, parents or other immediate family caretakers, extended family and community members, teachers, pediatricians, therapists, faith healers, the host culture, and the home culture [12]. These many vectors of influence form a complex but very rich web worth examining closely. There are many entities to juggle, and the process may at times be difficult [9]. If one respects context and remains curious, there is always rewarding work to be done in offering support to families in need.

The Complex Dynamics of Pharmacotherapy

The pharmacotherapist must be willing to dissect and explore the complex dynamics of prescribing and at times even give them voice when typically they might go unspoken by other stakeholders. An important starting place for consideration is the dynamics of power and authority [1]. When an immigrant child and their family present for psychiatric care, each member in the treatment alliance wields some important and particular powers. The youth patient holds the power of her symptoms and disclosure of relevant information. The parents hold the power to consent to the minor's treatment [5]. The clinicians hold the power of psychiatric diagnostic and treatment knowledge. Important questions include the following: In what manner does each individual wield that power? How do these powers intersect? How is authority balanced or imbalanced in the work together?

Now imagine that the pharmacotherapist recommends a psychiatric medication as possible clinical intervention. This might be considered a very authoritative position. That authority is instilled with a message which could be construed in different ways. Possible questions might arise about the message of the prescriber: Is that message one of hope, a sentiment that medication will be helpful? Or is it a message of doubt? Maybe even nonchalance? Each of these positions can have a significant impact on the treatment course and the effectiveness of selected interventions. The tone set by the pharmacotherapist is foundational for the remainder of the treatment process. Pumariega and colleagues [1] write, "culturally diverse families are more vulnerable to perceived or actual power differentials in their encounters with health care professionals" (p. 1103). This is worth acknowledging when working with immigrant families.

Another power dynamic is the power of *expectations*. The pharmacotherapist has expectations about the utility of the recommended medications. However, both the patient and parent and other stakeholders will have their own expectations about the potential impact of the medication. Consider whether these expectations are in alignment or whether they are distinct and differing among stakeholders.

Case Study: Medications and Assessing Expectations

Becca, a 14-year-old Salvadorian immigrant teenager, presents to the clinic with her father due to profound distress caused by worsening panic attacks that began post-migration. A child psychiatrist completes an intake interview and begins to develop a treatment plan that includes a recommendation for the patient to take a time-limited course of a benzodiazepine anxiolytic such as clonazepam. The psychiatrist hopes that this will decrease the frequency and intensity of her panic attacks. The adolescent seems excited about taking the benzodiazepine. When the psychiatrist inquires as to why, she says it is because she hopes the medication will "take away the anger I have about my parent's divorce." Upon seeking medication consent from the father, he also seems enthusiastic because he hopes "it will help put her to sleep at night. I hear she gets very upset at nights but I can never be there to console her because I work the night-shift for my job."

This case demonstrates that the stakeholders in this clinical interaction align in their support of the use of medications, but each for very different reasons. The pharmacotherapist can explore each person's expectations regarding the medication in order to shed light on his or her unique explanatory model of the panic attacks. Might discrepancies in these models and differential expectations regarding the medications undermine the treatment and its potential effectiveness? Will medication address the numerous psychosocial factors underlying this case?

Further discussion between the clinician, patient, and father leads to important reflections on this family's dynamics. The patient and father for the first time began to share with each other how divorce, distance from the mother, and financial strain had taken a toll on their relationship.

This case highlights the many nuances of authority, expectations, and hopes that can arise in the pharmacotherapy process. Interesting dynamics emerge as we think further about the role of the parent as a legal consenting adult in this and in any treatment scenario. It is not uncommon for feelings of guilt or anger to be present within the parent as related to their child's mental health circumstances [13]. As in this case, parents often feel a sense of responsibility for their child's symptoms. However, the opposite can also be true [14]. Some parents can have "psychological blind spots," such as being unaware of their own contribution to the child's struggles, even if it might be obvious to an outsider. Either of these psychological stances by a parent can have profound impact on perceptions that may develop about the role of medications in the treatment plan [5].

The parental role is an inherently multifaceted one. Regarding medications, the parental role can be as diverse as consenting, paying, administering, monitoring, or refilling the medications [11]. In addition, the parent may also have to take responsibility for managing any resistances that may arise if the child or adolescent at any time refuses to take the medication. This brings up important dynamics around autonomy that will be further explored later in the chapter.

Juggling all of these roles is a difficult task for any parent but can be particularly problematic for immigrant parents who have little prior contact with psychiatric medical culture. The pharmacotherapist can benefit from attunement to the parents' tolerance for that often unspoken psychiatric acculturation process and should always be curious about how the parents' own explanatory model of illness may differ from the medical model [15]. Unfamiliarity with the medical model might make some parents more comfortable with the pharmacotherapist being paternalistic in their clinical approach. On the other hand, unfamiliarity with the medical model might make some parents skeptical and averse to recommendations made by the pharmacotherapist [16, 17].

Case Study: Cross-Cultural Psychiatry—Medical vs. Nonmedical Models

Brenda, a 12-year-old *Mexican* girl who arrived in California 9 months ago, presents with her mother for clinical intake. The girl has been suffering with at least 6 months of severe mood symptoms. She is profoundly dysphoric with frequent tearful episodes, decreased interest in pleasurable activities, hopelessness, suicidality, self-harm behaviors, precipitous academic decline due to concentration impairment, limited energy, and poor sleep. The child psychiatrist does a comprehensive assessment including extensive discussions with the child, her mother, and the child's school teacher.

The physician meets in a follow-up visit with the mother and child and describes to them his belief that the child is experiencing a severe major depressive episode and would benefit from individual psychotherapy and treatment with an antidepressant such as fluoxetine. The child is hopeful that the medication could be helpful in relieving the incredible distress she has suffered over the better part of a year.

The physician asks the mother about the concerned look that has come over her face. The patient's mother goes on to say that she is considering consenting for the medication, but has quite a bit of ambivalence. She is unsure how helpful medications will be. She tells the physician that what the child really needs is an intervention based in a more "spiritual" approach informed by the strong religious foundation of their home community.

In this case, the patient, parent, and pharmacotherapist went on to have difficult but ultimately fruitful discussions about their varied explanatory models for her mood disturbance. The pharmacotherapist was inherently highly biologic in his formulation of the patient's depressive symptoms, and this differed significantly from the fundamentally spiritual conceptualization that the parent had. The pharmacotherapist discovered significant generational differences and varied influences of the immigration process on the parent and child.

Even at her relatively young age, the child had greater exposure to medical models of psychiatric care and expressed much more enthusiasm for the medication than her mother. The child went on to share that she enjoys aspects of her religious community but was very uncomfortable with the idea of participating in the religious ceremony that the patient's mother had been arranging for her at their place of worship. Ultimately they reached a compromise that the patient would take the medication and also meet with a youth group leader for spiritual support.

Pharmacotherapists should examine the messages brought into the pharmacotherapy space from the host culture and from the home culture about psychiatric diagnosis and medication treatment. What tensions or synergies exist at this interface? How do they impact the consenting parent and the suffering youth patient differently? Similarly?

Variations in Parental Involvement It should be noted how variable the definition of "parent" can be in immigrant families. There are a multitude of reasons why a child or their family might have left their homeland and immigrated. Therefore, it is not uncommon to discover that the child has a psychosocial issue with regard to their guardianship [18]. Issues might include one of the following: one or both of the child's biological parents are still back in the home country, the child has minimal contact with one or both biological parents, a parent is deceased, the child is living with extended family and their guardianship has been assumed by someone other than a biological parent, the child has never known one of their parents, or the child's parents are divorced [13, 19]. The demands of immigrant life can also make it very difficult for parents or guardians to be available to make frequent contact with clinicians. It is not uncommon for a teenage patient to show up to a follow-up appointment without their guardian due to the constraints of the parent's employment obligations or for other reasons. All of these variables can be challenging to manage in clinical settings. Pharmacotherapists should take time to investigate the family relationships influencing the immigrant youth patient and be prepared to understand how these relationships will impact any clinical decision-making that will be done around medications.

Medication and Its Psychological Meaning There are dynamic influences always at play when a pharmacotherapist contemplates the prescribing of a medication [4]. For any particular case, consider the following questions: What are the psychological processes at play within each stakeholder when a medication is prescribed? When is it not prescribed? When is a prescription accepted? When is a prescription declined? When is a medication prescribed, filled, and actually taken? When is a medication prescribed, filled, but not taken? Understanding the significance of the medication to the patient and their associated family system is paramount to the pharmacotherapist's conceptualization of the case.

Psychological meanings can be embedded in so many aspects of the pharmacotherapeutic process, including in how the actual medication itself is perceived. Clinicians should be curious about such meanings for our immigrant youth (Table 1). Pruett and colleagues [11] suggest exploring these meanings as they relate to the physical properties of the medication, the timing of administration, and who administers the medication.

Table 1 Possible meanings immigrant youth patients and/or their families might attribute to medication therapy

- This is a very big pill you have prescribed. That must mean it treats a very big problem. I hate feeling like there is a very big problem
- I'm so relieved. This medication is going to fix everything. And I hope it fixes it all very quickly
- This medication is going to fix nothing. It may even create more problems
- This pill represents a means of being controlled. It's like something is being "done to me"
- This medication might be dangerous. I heard that some medications are addictive
- I don't like the idea that I have to rely on a pill for me to be happier
- This medication proves that something serious has been going on. The seriousness of this situation has never otherwise felt validated until the medication was prescribed
- This medication confirms that there is something biological going on and that is a relief. We have no control over our biology. It's no-one's fault
- This medication confirms that there is something biological going on and that is horrible. Where did this biological problem come from? Whose fault is this?
- This medication reminds me that things are not "normal" the way we always hoped they would be
- This medication makes me feel different from everyone else. It makes me feel like people think there is something wrong with me. I guess there is something wrong with me
- Taking this medication will not be acceptable to my community
- Taking this medication has been extremely helpful to me and my family

It is also important to be aware that these meanings can shift over time in conjunction with the psychological development of the child and the family system. For example, a parent could initially feel resistant to the idea of their child being on an antidepressant and then over time become more willing to consider it after obtaining greater understanding from the pharmacotherapist. Or in the case of the meaning of side effects, weight gain associated with a medication can have very little meaning for a young child, but a very intense meaning for that same child at puberty when he or she is experiencing adolescent body preoccupation. Incremental appraisal of these meanings over the course of treatment can reveal these shifts in meaning as they happen [20].

Psychiatric medications are most effective when they are actually taken by the patient. Diligent adherence to the prescribed medication can better ensure more rapid and complete remission of symptoms. This is especially crucial in cases involving severe mental illness, like psychotic states and/or severe mood disordered states where delusions, suicidality, aggression, or other forms of agitation can not only profoundly compromise functionality, but could risk the life of the patient or others [21]. Not uncommonly, ambivalent patients and families will behaviorally express their internal uncertainty about psychiatric care through intermittent medication adherence or even complete nonadherence [22]. Pharmacotherapists might consider this a sign that more exploration is required regarding the patient and family's level of commitment to medication use. To improve adherence, it can be helpful to work with the patient and family to review the treatment course and draw links between periods of functional decompensation with periods of nonadherence [11].

There are many misconceptions about psychiatric medications. A very common misconception has been described as "the delusion of precision," a phrase coined by Gutheil [23]. This is the notion that "drugs are specific, concrete, targeted agents, that are uniformly effective as long as a doctor prescribes them" (Gutheil [23], p. 322). Even if fundamentally false, this could be experienced as a primary hope and tenet carrying psychological meaning for a parent or patient who accepts a medication prescription from a pharmacotherapist. This principle can apply to other stakeholders in the child's well-being such as school teachers or administrators. It is important to respect the hope that often grows within the treatment alliance once a medication is prescribed. However, it is also necessary for pharmacotherapists to acknowledge to self and others the limits of medication. Very rarely is medication efficacy as precise as stakeholders wish.

Countertransference Just as in psychotherapy, effective pharmacotherapy requires the clinician to be very self-aware. Elements of countertransference will be present in the act of medication prescribing. Self-examination questions for a psychopharmocologist include: When do I have the urge to prescribe, where is that urge coming from? Am I responding to an internal pressure to "do something"? How much external pressure do I feel from the family, the school, etc.? When I have the urge not to prescribe, what forces are contributing to my hesitation? The clinician may ask himself or herself, when does pharmacotherapy feel like an onerous enterprise? When do I most enjoy it? How do I feel when a patient or family is ambivalent about medications? How do I feel when a patient or family seems to have unreasonable expectations of the pharmacotherapy being offered? How do I feel when a patient or family seems naïve, unaware, or limited in their psychological mindedness? As I write this prescription, am I feeling like it will bring me closer to this patient or family? Or will it distance me from them? The more comfortable the pharmacotherapist can become with asking these questions and observing the internal patterns that may arise, the more effective a pharmacotherapist will be in understanding his/her role in the dynamic.

Patient Autonomy and the Pharmacotherapeutic Process

Medication prescribing for immigrant youth populations both reveals and engages very complex dynamics of family and culture. The issue of *autonomy* is one that frequently arises as a necessary area of exploration in the pharmacotherapeutic process. Autonomy in the context of the practice of medicine often refers to the right of the patient to make informed decisions free of coercion. When working with children and adolescents, the nuances of autonomy become very salient influences in the therapeutic alliance. It is the guardians of the minor that have the right to consent to medications, and not the child/adolescent themselves! [4].

Case Study: Autonomy and Medication Administration

Ali, a 10-year-old Eritrean immigrant boy, presents for psychiatric evaluation. He has a multitude of symptoms consistent with combined-type ADHD and would likely benefit from a stimulant medication to treat it. Both his school life and home life are being compromised due to marked inattention, hyperactivity, and impulsivity.

His aunt and uncle (legal guardians) are extremely invested in securing a medication prescription for their nephew. They are hopeful that the appropriate medication would assist him in becoming a more successful student, especially as he enters the more academically intensive middle school years. His guardians state, "All we want is for him to be able to learn so that he can get a good job and live a better life than we have. And his bad behavior in the classroom is drawing too much negative attention to our family!" The pharmacotherapist prescribes methylphenidate (a stimulant) to be taken by the patient each morning, and the aunt and uncle enthusiastically give consent.

From the beginning, the patient himself expressed dissent. Regarding his preference not to be medicated, he states, "I really don't want to be controlled by that pill!" In protest, he begins to refuse to take the pill. Out of desperation, his aunt and uncle begin to secretly crush the pills and slip them into his breakfast each morning. The aunt and uncle reveal this to the pharmacotherapist in a follow-up appointment. They hoped to get the clinician's blessing to continue the current mode of secret medication administration.

Some caregivers will feel compelled to conceal the medication from the child. As in this case, it may be because the child refuses to take the medication. In other cases, it may be because the caregiver wants to "protect" the child and does not want them to know they need medication. When a pharmacotherapist discovers that there is covert activity arising that compromises the autonomy of the patient, it is important to explore these dynamics.

The pharmacotherapist should approach this situation with curiosity, exploration, and respect of context, as these are the guiding principles of pharmacotherapy. However, the clinician could feel inclined to discourage surreptitious behavior, and more often than not this stance is reasonable. Though the caregiver's intentions can be sympathized with, supporting the autonomy of the child is usually well worth it in these situations.

If the patient discovers that they have been tricked into taking medications, there is a high risk that the child will become hostile and distrusting toward the caregiver and possibly the physician as well. Supporting autonomy and discouraging deceit protects these critical family relationships, protects the alliance between physician and child, as well as protects the long-term trust the child will have for the greater institution of mental health care. Ideally, pharmacotherapy will be as transparent as possible in order to safeguard these relationships.

Alliances The management of the family dynamics as they unfold in the above case reveals an interesting element of the pharmacotherapeutic experience—the potential for suballiances to form within the treatment alliance [5]. We like to think of the clinician, patient, and caregivers as aligned in an ideal treatment alliance. The realities are inevitably much more complicated. A suballiance can occur when there is a merger between select parties in the treatment alliance around particular issues to the exclusion of other stakeholders. As in the above case, the caregivers had formed a suballiance around medication administration and were hoping to recruit the pharmacotherapist into that suballiance, though not with any obvious malicious intent.

A strong argument can be made that the pharmacotherapist is first and foremost in suballiance with their child or adolescent patient. It is that child who is being asked to ingest prescribed medication. It is that vulnerable child who often bears the weight of the family pathology and the complex cultural dynamics. It is the job of the pharmacotherapist to advocate for the child given this level of vulnerability. This can conflict with a parent's hope that the pharmacotherapist will act primarily as an emissary of the parental agenda. The clinician must be attuned to this challenging aspect of the work [5].

There are also more subtle ways that parental agendas can begin to supersede the autonomy of the child. Parents bring their own preconceptions about psychiatric care (whether positive, skeptical, or neutral) to the table as decisions are being made about their child's care. These preconceptions may be based on what they have heard from others in their community or from their own personal experience with psychiatric care. These are powerful messages that are carried into the pharmacotherapeutic treatment space as parents consider medicating their child. Sometimes these messages can be far more influential than the seeming authority of the pharmacotherapist themselves. These preconceptions must be examined critically alongside the parent so that an informed conclusion can be made as to how influential the preconception should be in the decision-making around the mental health of the child. The goal is not necessarily to eradicate the preconceptions as much as it is to ensure that they do not go unexamined [5].

Case Study: Working with Unfavorable Impressions of Psychiatric Care

Paula, a 16-year-old Colombian immigrant girl, presents for evaluation of panic with agoraphobia. Her frequent and severe panic episodes are contributing to significant functional decline including occasional school refusal at this critical time in her high school career. She is concerned that she will not be able to fulfill her dream of matriculating at a competitive 4-year college.

The pharmacotherapist strongly recommends psychotherapy for this teenage patient. However, the clinician also suggests that in addition she may benefit from initiation of an antidepressant medication for treatment of anxiety. She reviews the risks, benefits, and alternatives. The teenager is hopeful that this can be a helpful adjunct to psychotherapy.

However, her adult sister (legal guardian) is hesitant to consent for the medication. The pharmacotherapist begins to inquire about the source of her hesitation. The sister reveals that as a child, she herself was placed on a stimulant medication for treatment of ADHD, and it was a "terrible experience." She describes that it caused her appetite suppression, insomnia, palpitations, and agitation and she discontinued the medication after a few weeks. The sister explains "It was really hard for me to bring her to a psychiatrist because ever since my experience when I was younger I haven't really trusted psychiatry. I don't want her to go through what I went through. It was so terrible. I don't want her on medication."

The pharmacotherapist listened attentively to the sister's concerns and validated the suffering she had experienced as a child on medication. She also affirmed that these experiences will undoubtedly come to bear on the current circumstance where the sister was witnessing her loved one's level of distress and wishing no further distress on her in the form of medication side effects. The pharmacotherapist took the time to revisit a discussion of the risks and benefits of antidepressants as well as to distinguish them from stimulants in indication, mechanism, and side effect profile.

An important area of clarification was to inform the sister that the patient would need to take the antidepressant every day to get optimal benefit and for several weeks before benefits might be detectable. The sister disclosed that she had hoped the medication could still be effective if taken only once or twice a week so as to minimize potential side effects. The pharmacotherapist helped the sister to understand that antidepressants are not best taken intermittently or as needed in the way that stimulants can be. The pharmacotherapist was pleased to clarify this so as to avoid future adherence issues.

The clinician spent time examining with the guardian what aspects of her teenage sister's clinical situation were similar and unique from her own. The teenage patient also spent some time sharing with her sister why she desired to take the medication. The guardian acknowledged that she had heavily conflated her own history with that of her anxious teen sister.

Though she was not prepared to consent for the medication immediately, the sister proposed the following compromise: she agreed that her anxious sister should begin psychotherapy as soon as possible. She requested that an appointment be set with the pharmacotherapist 4 weeks from now. She hoped by that time she would have done further research on the proposed medication and have a better sense how effective the therapy alone might be for the patient.

When the patient and her sister returned for follow-up, they revealed that after extensive family discussion, they had decided to move forward with the medication. The patient saw much improvement with a combination of cognitive behavioral therapy and medication.

Thoughtful discussion is useful when the consenting adult's perceptions of psychiatric care are unfavorable as in the previous case but also when perceptions are favorable. This is illustrated in the below case:

Case Study: Working with Favorable Impressions of Psychiatric Care

Vinh is a 15-year-old Vietnamese immigrant boy with history of ADHD well controlled on atomoxetine who presents to a pharmacotherapist for evaluation of depression. He has been in psychotherapy for several months, and his therapist has referred him to a child psychiatrist for consideration of adjunctive medication. After extensive assessment, the child psychiatrist agrees that the patient could benefit from antidepressant medication.

The patient and his mother agreed with the recommendation to initiate an antidepressant. To the pharmacotherapist's surprise, the mother makes a request for a very specific medication. She is particularly invested in her child being prescribed fluoxetine (a commonly used antidepressant). The clinician inquires as to why, and the mother shares that a child in their immediate cultural community who is a family friend had also been suffering from depression. She had spoken to that child's mother and she had shared that a psychiatric evaluation and prescription for fluoxetine had really provided great improvement for that child and the family.

The pharmacotherapist noticed his own relief in recognizing that he would not have to do much to convince this parent that the child could benefit from a medication. In this case, the patient's home community seemed to support the family in their decision. However, the pharmacotherapist was very concerned about the mother's specific medication request. The pharmacotherapist had noticed in his time as a physician that he often becomes frustrated when a parent attempts to dictate care. He quickly noted that in this case he would need to be vigilant for this potential countertransference.

He also was uncomfortable for more purely biologic reasons. The patient is on atomoxetine for ADHD, and this medication is known to have a concerning drug-drug interaction with the requested antidepressant, fluoxetine. This drug-drug interaction is less prominent with other antidepressant medications in the selective-serotonin-reuptake-inhibitor class including escitalopram or citalopram. The pharmacotherapist felt comfortable with either of these agents as an alternative to fluoxetine.

The patient's mother felt frustration that the pharmacotherapist declined to prescribe fluoxetine. After extensive discussion, she expressed understanding as to why a trial of fluoxetine would carry risk of compromise to patient's health in a fashion that was avoidable and difficult to justify. The pharmacotherapist presented escitalopram and citalopram (other antidepressants) as alternatives to the mother who was grateful to have a choice of agents, if fluoxetine could not be initiated. The pharmacotherapist carefully reviewed the risks and benefits of each medication with the family. He also noted the risk and benefits associated with declining treatment altogether, as he does in any consent process. The mother ultimately selected escitalopram because she felt her son could benefit from treatment and because escitalopram specifically carries an FDA indication for treatment of depression in adolescents just as does fluoxetine.

Developmental Shifts and Autonomy Autonomy can also refer to the level of direct involvement the patient has in his or her own care. This can shift over the developmental spectrum [24]. For example, a young child will typically have a limited capacity to integrate all of the complex data that goes into making a clinical decision. On the other hand, many adolescents can both synthesize this data and speak articulately about whether or not they would like to take medication and even specify which one, based on the information at hand. It is critical that pharmacotherapists seek the adolescent's assent in prescribing a medication, though it is the caregiving adult who has the final legal authority to consent [5].

The pharmacotherapist must always assess what the patient's level of developmental maturity is. This assessment is an ongoing process because the patient will likely be observed progressing in their maturity longitudinally [25]. The pharmacotherapist can be encouraging increased ownership and input by the young patient in the pharmacotherapy experience over time but always appropriate to developmental level [5].

Combined Versus Collaborative Pharmacotherapy

In the opening of the chapter, the "bicultural" expression of the pharmacotherapist was discussed. The term "bicultural" here denotes a clinician fluent in both the psychological and the biological. This clinical ability is essential in the case of caring for immigrant children. The pharmacotherapist must employ his psychological knowledge even around the intricately dynamic act of medication prescribing. However, the pharmacotherapist will also need to determine if they would like to formally take on the role of psychotherapist, meeting consistently with the client in psychotherapy sessions.

Formally combining the role of pharmacotherapist with the role of psychotherapist within the same clinician can be a very effective and integrative treatment model. It can truly enhance a clinician's knowledge of the patient, family, and their cultural background. It gives a better sense of whether medications can be helpful. Very rarely is a medication alone enough to offer comprehensive treatment for a psychological problem. The combined pharmacotherapist/psychotherapist will have the wherewithal to offer therapeutic intervention in areas where the medication may be able to offer symptom relief but may not reach the fundamental source of a child's struggle.

There are certainly circumstances where treatment will need to be split such that the pharmacotherapist and the psychotherapist are two distinct clinicians.

Sometimes the structure of the medical system mandates these roles be delegated to different clinicians. Sometimes the best-fit therapist based on an essential factor like language capability is not a prescribing mental health professional. Sometimes split treatment is appropriate when medication concerns are complex enough that spending the necessary time on discussing meds would threaten the time needed to fully engage the psychotherapy process. Mental health care with a pharmacologist and a separate psychotherapist is referred to as "split treatment," but the spirit is more accurately one of collaborative care [26].

In collaborative treatment, clinicians must be highly communicative with each other [27]. Each must make efforts to remain highly informed about and engaged in the arm of treatment that they are not directly responsible for. Medications can carry profound meaning for patients and their families. The mere presence of medications within the treatment plan often has important impact on the patient and family's therapeutic engagement. For example, the presence of medications can relieve symptoms to the extent that the patient is more open to engage in therapy. In other instances, the presence of medications can make a patient or their caregivers feel as if psychotherapy is redundant. These are the sorts of issues that must be explored by both the pharmacotherapist and the psychotherapist together as they discuss their impressions of the case over time and explored by each clinician with the patient themselves.

Special Issues in Pharmacotherapy of Immigrant Populations

Critical Appraisal of the Literature The number of pediatric psychopharmacology trials is limited. When dealing with unique populations, such as that of immigrant pediatric cases, the issue of research conclusion generalizability often arises. Medication trials rarely include subjects that reflect the full cultural diaspora [1]. With that in mind, the pharmacotherapist must be prepared to discover unique treatment experiences that are not always comprehensively reflected in the literature [28].

Ethnopsychopharmacology Ethnopsychopharmacology refers to the growing literature and practice of recognizing that variations exist in the human response to psychiatric medications across racial and ethnic lines [29]. Pharmacotherapists working with immigrant youth populations should become familiar with principles of ethnopsychopharmacology [1]. The knowledge that differences exist in pharmacokinetics and pharmacodynamics based on heritable genetic variants that affect cultural communities can help us anticipate differential outcomes [20].

Complementary and Alternative Medicine (CAM) Patients and families with connections to non-Western healing traditions may choose to incorporate into the treatment regimen complementary and alternative medication (CAM) agents or other interventions such as dietary modifications [20]. Pharmacotherapists should be prepared to inquire about these and explore the meanings infused in these treatments for the patient and family [30]. Familiarity with alternative medications is helpful for pharmocotherapists. The pharmacotherapist must be prepared to educate herself about them as she discovers the patient is using them. Just as in the inquiry around any other medication, it is important for the pharmocotherapist to understand the hope that the patient and family have with regard to the contribution of these CAM agents to the treatment plan. The pharmacotherapist must consider not only the possible biologic drug-drug interactions, but also his/her own cultural attitude toward Western medicine versus alternative treatments. Typically, pharmacotherapists trained in an allopathic tradition will make allopathic-style recommendations. If a family is more comfortable with herbal treatments, the tensions that exist at this cultural juncture between allopathic and herbal medicine should be explored with humility [1].

Finances and Language Regarding additional pragmatics of prescribing for immigrant families, the pharmacotherapist must consider issues such as financial means and language [17]. Choose medications appropriate to the patient's clinical needs but in addition remain informed by what the family's financial resources are. In child psychiatry, there are typically affordable pharmaceutical options that are equally as effective as their more costly counterparts [10]. As part of the practice of dynamic exploration in pharmacotherapy, the clinician should reflect with the patient and family on any concerns about how financial means will impact quality of care. These are often very real, honest, authentic concerns that must be acknowledged in order to build a trusting treatment alliance. If appropriate and available, the pharmocotherapist should try to provide written materials about medications or any other aspects of treatment in the family's primary language. Language interpreters are integral members of the clinical care team and should be utilized during appointments whenever possible [1] (Table 2).

Table 2 Clinical pearls for pharmacotherapy with immigrant families

• Take the time to be thorough in assessment and to appreciate that the psychosocial situation with its cultural influences can be very fluid. An appreciation of this fluid backdrop is essential for employing medications most appropriately, if at all.
• The formulation should precede the prescription [11].
• Be prepared to offer as much education and knowledge as possible, so that patient and family feel informed about the medication treatments being offered or employed. Pace this appropriately to the needs of the family.
• Restore hope and infuse a sense of future wherever possible [11].
• The treatment stance should always be one of understanding. Be curious about the many perspectives that will be at play in the pharmacotherapy treatment space. Be prepared to negotiate discrepancies in perspective.

References

1. Pumariega AJ, Rothe E, Mian A, Carlisle L, Toopelberg C, Harris T, et al. The American Academy of child and adolescent psychiatry (AACAP) committee on quality issues (CQI): practice parameter for cultural competence in child and adolescent psychiatric practice. J Am Acad Child Adolesc Psychiatry. 2013;52(10):1101–15.
2. Toppelberg C, Collins B. Language, culture, and adaptation in immigrant children. Child Adolesc Psychiatr Clin N Am. 2010;19(4):697–717.
3. Pumariega AJ, Joshi SV. Culture and development in children and youth. Child Adolesc Psychiatr Clin N Am. 2010;19(4):661–80.
4. Dell ML, et al. Ethics and the prescription pad. Child Adolesc Psychiatr Clin N Am. 2008;17(1):93–111.
5. Joshi SV. Teamwork: the therapeutic alliance in pediatric pharmacotherapy. Child Adolesc Psychiatr Clin N Am. 2006;15(1):239–62.
6. Storck MG, Vander SA. Fostering ecologic perspectives in child psychiatry. Child Adolesc Psychiatr Clin N Am. 2007;16(1):133–63.
7. Gabbard G, Kay J. The fate of integrated treatment: whatever happened to the biopsychosocial psychiatrist? Am J Psychiatr. 2001;158:1956–63.
8. Kleinman A, Eisenberg L, Good B. Culture, illness, and care: clinical lessons from anthropological and cross-cultural research. Ann Intern Med. 1978;88:251–88.
9. Aggarwal N. Cultural formulations in child and adolescent psychiatry. J Am Acad Child Adolesc Psychiatry. 2010;49(4):306–9.
10. Kouyoumdjian H, et al. Barriers to community mental health services for Latinos: treatment considerations. Clin Psychol Sci Pract. 2003;10(4):394–422.
11. Pruett KP, Joshi SV, Martin A. Thinking about prescribing: the psychology of psychopharmacology. In: Martin A, Scahill L, Kratochvil C, editors. Pediatric psychopharmacology: principles and practice. 2nd ed. New York, NY: Oxford University Press; 2010. p. 422–34.
12. Pumariega A, et al. Culturally informed child psychiatric practice. Child Adolesc Psychiatr Clin N Am. 2010;19(4):739–57.
13. Walsh F. Traumatic loss and major disasters: strengthening family and community resilience. Family Process. 2007;46(2):207–27.
14. Choi H. Understanding adolescent depression in ethnocultural context. Adv Nurs Sci. 2002;25(2):71–85.
15. Pumariega A, Rothe E. Leaving no children or families behind: the challenges of immigration. Am J Orthopsychiatr. 2010;80(4):505–15.
16. Rothe E, Tzuang D, Pumariega A. Acculturation, development, and adaptation. Child Adolesc Psychiatr Clin N Am. 2010;19(4):681–96.
17. Alegria M, Vallas M, Pumariega A. Racial and ethnic disparities in pediatric mental health. Child Adolesc Psychiatr Clin N Am. 2010;19(4):759–74.
18. Suarez-Orozco C, et al. Growing up in the shadows: the developmental implications of unauthorized status. Harv Educ Rev. 2011;81(3):438–72.
19. Suarez-Orozco C, et al. Making up for last time: the experience of separation and reunification among immigrant families. Fam Process. 2002;41(4):625–43.
20. Malik M. Culturally adapted pharmacotherapy and the integrative formulation. Child Adolesc Psychiatr Clin N Am. 2010;19(4):791–814.
21. Balan I, Moyers T, Lewis-Fernandez R. Motivational pharmacotherapy: combining motivational interviewing and antidepressant therapy to improve treatment adherence. Psychiatry. 2013;76(3):203–9.
22. Cromer B, Tarnowski K. Noncompliance in adolescents: a review. J Dev Behav Pediatr. 1989;10(4):207–15.
23. Gutheil T. The psychology of psychopharmacology. Bull Menninger Clin. 1982;46:321–30.
24. Kwak K. Adolescents and their parents: a review of intergenerational family relations for immigrant and non-immigrant families. Hum Dev. 2003;46(2–3):115–36.

25. Titzmann P. Growing up too soon? Parentification among immigrant and native adolescents in Germany. J Youth Adolesc. 2012;41(7):880–93.
26. Sederer L, et al. Guidelines for prescribing psychiatrists in consultative, collaborative, and supervisory relationships. Psychiatr Serv. 1998;49(9):1197–202.
27. Feinstein N, et al. The supporting alliance in child and adolescent treatment: enhancing collaboration among therapists, parents, and teachers. Am J Psychother. 2009;63(4):319–44.
28. Pi E, Simpson G. Cross-cultural psychopharmacology: a current clinical perspective. Psychiatr Serv. 2005;56(1):31–3.
29. Chaudry IB, et al. Ethnicity and psychopharmacology. J Psychopharmacol. 2008;22(6): 673–80.
30. Kemper K, et al. The use of complementary and alternative medicine in pediatrics. Pediatrics. 2008;122(6):1374–86.

Information Systems and Technology

Eduardo Bunge, Megan K. Jones, Benjamin Dickter,
Rosaura Perales, and Andrea Spear

*Adapting paper and pencil face-to-face psychotherapy
procedures to meet the demands of the virtual and digital
revolution paves the way forward.*

Friedberg et al. [1]

Abstract

Immigrant youths often struggle with a variety of mental and physical challenges associated with moving to a new country. These challenges can be adaptively confronted through digital communication and information technology (CIT) particularly for those who are digitally native and capable of navigating electronic systems. This chapter first defines the ways in which CIT can increase the reach and capability of psychotherapy when working with immigrant youth and, finally, an exploration of the potential risks and ethical issues, which may develop when these interventions are provided. ·

Keywords

Immigrant youth • Digital native generation • Communication and information technology • Psychotherapy

Introduction

Digital technologies can aid both immigrant youth and the hosting nation in facing the problems associated with immigration. Psychotherapy for immigrant youth can exploit the global development of communication and information technology (CIT), which has resulted in a worldwide digital native generation: those born among technology and comfortable with navigating such systems [2]. There is a wide variety of evidence-based treatment for anxiety, depression, and behavioral problems of youth using digital technology (e.g., [1, 3–9]). Additionally, the most

E. Bunge (✉) • M.K. Jones • B. Dickter • R. Perales • A. Spear
Palo Alto University, 1791 Arastradero Road, Palo Alto, CA 94304, USA
e-mail: ebunge@paloaltou.edu

© Springer International Publishing Switzerland 2016
S.G. Patel, D. Reicherter (eds.), *Psychotherapy for Immigrant Youth*,
DOI 10.1007/978-3-319-24693-2_7

predicted innovations for therapy in the coming years include increased use of online self-help therapies, smartphone applications, virtual reality, and social networking interventions [10]. However, to date there are no studies focusing on the implementation of these treatments in populations of immigrant youth. This chapter is intended to offer suggestions for clinicians seeking to engage immigrant youth in therapy via CIT.

This chapter will define CIT, the ways in which youth across the globe interact with it, and how immigrant youth can benefit from the global access of CIT. This will be followed with a discussion of ways in which CIT can augment psychotherapy, including hypothetical case examples, and potential ethical issues when introducing such systems to immigrant youth.

Immigrant Youth and Communication and Information Technology

Youth who were born after 1995 are known as "Generation Z" or "the Millennials" [11]. This generation is often described as "digitally native," having grown up in a hyper-connected world where technology is pervasive. Technology is continuously evolving and creating new methods of communication that are widely used by clients in their everyday lives and can be included in psychotherapy. In general, CIT includes devices such as radios, televisions, telephones, cameras, computers, tablets, software applications, video cameras, video games, and any other interactive modes of communication [12].

The ways in which immigrant youth can access the Internet impact the usefulness of Internet interventions [13]. The "digital divide" is a term used to define the differences in access and use of the Internet across cultural and socioeconomic boundaries [14, 15, 16]. While originally defined solely through access, where racial minorities, low socioeconomic status individuals, and rural communities had a significantly lower ability to use and interact with web-based technologies [17], the use of Internet-connected devices have become more ubiquitous, and a significant difference in the use of Internet technologies across various groups has emerged. Those with a higher source of income and higher levels of education often use the Internet for personal growth opportunities, for example, as an educational tool. Those with lower socioeconomic statuses have been found to use the Internet mainly for entertainment and socialization purposes, limiting the benefits of an information-rich World Wide Web [13]. Another factor that impacts a person's ability to understand and effectively make use of the Internet is the ability to speak English [18]. Homes of immigrants, where English is not the spoken language, have much lower access and usage rates of the Internet, leading to fewer resources for career opportunities and other areas of adaptation. The digital divide imitates inequality from the real world, in which English ability and racial influences can greatly impact a person's functioning in society [19].

Despite the discrepancies in Internet usage, state and local governments have increased Internet access to the public through the library system [20, 21]. The

United States library system is capable of offering Internet access to those who either cannot or will not acquire means of access at home. As such, the American government has increased the number of services available online, using librarians as first-stop disseminators of information regarding such services [20]. The utilization of libraries to access information, both public and private, on the Internet has increased greatly in the last decade, with natives and immigrants using library computers at equal rates [18]. Because technology surrounding Internet access is advancing at rapid rates, such access will likely reach near saturation in the coming year (for a more in depth discussion about immigration resources, see chapter "Immigrant Youth and Navigating Unique Systems of Treatment").

Youth coupled with immigration brings about significant emotional, behavioral, and cognitive difficulties [22–24]. However, immigration can foster personal growth if enough internal and external resources are available to assist in a successful transition [25]. Recent research has found that mass media serves as an important source in adaption for immigrant youth [26–28] (Durham, 2004 as cited in Elias and Lemish [29]). More specifically, research shows that the Internet is used as a way to provide adolescents with the resources for identity construction [30, 31].

For example, immigrant youth with a deep sense of loss may use the Internet to "reinvent" their homeland [29]. Through native country Web pages, youths are able to control the frequency and intensity of their relationship with the virtual form of their home country, which in turn provides coping resources during a time of profound insecurity and vulnerability. It has also been found that online chat rooms and messaging programs provide young immigrants the opportunity to form interpersonal connections with co-ethnic peers [29]. In this sense, immigrant youths use the Internet as a form of coping with the loneliness that is characteristic during migration. These chat rooms also act as virtual support networks that can assist young immigrants facing major challenges. Besides providing immigrant youth with meaningful interpersonal connections, the Internet is used as a way to learn about the new host country. Host country websites are common among young immigrants as a way to gain knowledge of cultural customs and traditions [29]. Overall, the Internet plays a large role in the identity construction of immigrant youth by providing them with the ability to experience multiple cultures at once [29]. In addition, because it allows for anonymous communications, the Internet offers a unique vehicle for identity exploration, allowing for free expression of emotions and the maturation of intimate relationships [32, 33].

Immigrant youths are susceptible to many challenges in their new host country. A common theme that appears among most immigrants is stress related to exclusion, poverty, and separation [34]. Practitioners working with immigrant youth should consider the possibility of using social media as a helpful tool, as the digital world can influence self-appraisal in a positive way [35]. The social media networks of the digital world can help immigrants stay in contact with their family and friends from their home country. Social media is used more than any other source for interacting with other individuals [36], with Facebook reporting over 829 million active users [37]. Social media impact how immigrant youths think, feel, and behave as they compare themselves to other individuals [36]. These comparisons may increase self-esteem for those who post positive stories and receive more encouraging comments [38]. Conversely, youth may experience decreased self-esteem related to awareness of personal "limitations and shortcomings" [35, p. 1], which has been linked to mood and anxiety disorders [39, 40]. Despite the negative social comparisons, Facebook provides users with resources for numerous help groups when faced with challenging emotions or feelings of negative social disconnect which can increase feelings of community and belonging. Social media outlets allow individuals to compare ideas, voice opinions, share thoughts, and receive commentary feedback on social views. At this time, further research is needed on the effectiveness of incorporating the social media of Facebook groups into the therapeutic system.

While the role of CIT is increasing in the lives of immigrant youth, it is important to consider the limitations associated with this dissemination. As stated above, a considerable digital divide exists between types of usage across socioeconomic groups. These differences, combined with the heavy bias towards Western civilizations and the English language within the Internet may hamper an immigrant youth's ability to engage in CIT interventions.

Communication and Information Technology Resources in Psychotherapy

Although the importance of youth mental health and the prevention of disorders are widely recognized, a large gap remains between those seeking help and the resources available to them [41]. From a professional perspective, the resources available to treat those seeking treatment are inherently limited. Traditional interventions require high therapist-to-client ratios in order for psychotherapy to occur, a disadvantage not shared by CIT-based treatments [42]. However, immigrant youths frequently lack the knowledge or ability to access mental health and immigration resources through digital technology [43].

Advances in intervention delivery through technology will result in enormous contributions to mental and physical health and well-being [44]. Mental health resources using CIT can be used either alone or in session with a therapist. These resources can be integrated into face-to-face psychotherapy, incorporate specific programs known as computer-aided psychotherapy, be used as an adjunct to therapist-delivered treatment, introduce telepsychotherapy, or even provide self-automated online help. Clinical applications that accompany technological advances allow clinicians to reach clients beyond the provision of "brick and mortar" services [44].

Regarding the use of CIT in psychotherapy, Friedberg et al. [1] highlighted several reasons in favor of the utilization of smartphones, computers, and other devices by those who practice cognitive behavioral therapy (CBT). Providing psychotherapy via emerging technologies changes the method of service delivery [1]. Through the use of smartphone applications (apps), video games, and computer programs, therapy may become more engaging to youth because of their similarity to

Table 1 Different levels of technology use in psychotherapy

Type of therapy	Definition	Amount of client-therapist contact	Example intervention
Face-to-face psychotherapy	Consisting of one-on-one treatment with a therapist that may include technology to increase contact	++	Telepsychotherapy
Digital psychotherapy	Consisting face-to-face therapies combined with digital interventions	+	Camp cope-a-lot
Digital self-help	Primarily consisting of technology as a main intervention with minimal interaction with a therapist	−	BRAVE

++ Considerable amount of client-therapist contact; + moderate amount of client-therapist contact; − absence of client-therapist contact

entertainment devices [45], such as mainstream video games and handheld entertainment systems. In particular, smartphones are portable, accessible, widely used, programmable, unobtrusive, and contain sophisticated graphic, video, audio, photographic, and text capabilities [46]. Smartphones are currently being used in everyday life, and as technology moves to increasingly capable phones, intervention possibilities increase as well [44]. As an example of such new technology, video games capture youth interests and increase engagement in therapy, in the way board games have in the past. In addition, video games offer advantages over board games such as increased opportunity to practice "frustration tolerance, cooperation, proper communication, and memory/attention" skills [1, p. 10].

The integration of digital technology in psychotherapy can range from face-to-face sessions with minimal technology along a spectrum to digital self-help as shown in Table 1. Face-to-face psychotherapy/telepsychotherapy consists of sessions where the therapist works one-on-one with a client using minimal means of technology. Digital psychotherapy exists as a spectrum in which face-to-face therapy and digital interventions that do not require direct therapist guidance combine to form a cohesive treatment. Digital self-help consists of primarily using technologies such as smartphone applications and online websites, with no intervention from a therapist. (For more information on these specific topics, please see content under specified headings.)

Integrating Technology to Face-to-Face Psychotherapy

Psychotherapy, regardless of theoretical orientation or intervention type, involves a range of techniques used to increase client well-being. These techniques can be augmented using CIT in a variety of ways. The following are examples of how to use CIT in order to build rapport, increase understanding in psychoeducation, aid in relaxation techniques, increase exposure effectiveness, and help in relapse prevention. Hypothetical case examples are used to show methods of interacting with immigrant youth, exploiting the unique advantages offered by CIT-related interventions.

Building Rapport

Building rapport with youth in therapy is essential in developing a trusting relationship where the client feels comfortable talking openly with his or her therapist [47]. Adding CIT to therapy helps develop strong bonds with youth, increase motivation, and develop respect and trust between client and therapist [45]. CIT may provide a useful resource in developing rapport with immigrant youth, who are members of "Generation Z" and were born into a computerized, Internet-connected world [11]. Friedberg and colleagues [1] mention that traditionally therapists used board games to build rapport with children but that such a task can be adapted for the modern generation with video games. Video games may help youth to attend sessions both more regularly and actively, increase satisfaction with their treatment, enhance motivation for child psychotherapy, and strengthen the relationship with the therapist [4, 48]. Elliott [49] specifically highlights the game Minecraft (a game where players get unlimited resources to build a world of their own) as a way of engaging adolescents in an atypical manner that can allow them to learn skills such as the ability to self-define goals in an open world format. Other methods of developing rapport include using the Internet in a collaborative way to understand the client's culture and viewing the client's old neighborhood together through satellite mapping websites.

The following is an example of ways to use CIT to build rapport with an immigrant youth:

Case Study

Yugi is a 15-year-old Japanese male who immigrated to San Francisco Bay Area with his parents one month ago. Despite having learned English at a young age and being top of his class in Japan, Yugi is struggling in school due to depressive symptoms. In Japan, Yugi lived with many of his extended relatives, including both pairs of grandparents, aunts, uncles, and three cousins close to Yugi's age. He often played outside in his neighborhood and with video games with cousins and friends. Using CIT, Yugi's therapist has several different options for establishing rapport with him.

One way in which the therapist developed rapport and learned about Yugi's cultural perspective involved using the Internet. Cultural artifacts from Japan, such as favorite music or television shows, were found on video sharing sites as a way to show the therapist different aspects of Yugi's life. He also showed his family's house, neighborhood, and favorite parts of the city on a map, broadening discussion beyond the computer screen. The therapist enhanced the therapeutic alliance with Yugi by incorporating video games into sessions. Minecraft was used within therapy to facilitate the interaction with the therapist, promoting an increase in participant engagement during sessions and increasing the frequency of session attendance. Specifically, the therapist and Yugi worked in a collaborative way using the Minecraft metaphor to define the steps needed to achieve his goals. Additionally, the therapist and client worked together in creating, through Minecraft, a world that contains different components from both his native culture and American culture.

Psychoeducation

Psychoeducation of a mental health disorder before beginning therapy is an important element to further help the youth and the parent understand the symptoms, triggers, and resources available to improve symptoms [50]. Therapists may be able to engage youth and parents to increase knowledge and awareness of mental health disorders by providing psychoeducation materials through different forms of technology including smartphone applications, informative podcasts, online psychoeducation, and CD-ROMS.

Smartphone applications can engage youth and provide information on specific diagnoses and associated symptoms through a user-friendly format [8]. Additionally, podcasts are becoming more readily available as a way to stream informative psychoeducation audio recordings about topics like specific disorders. Podcasts are easily accessible and can be used at an individual's convenience [5]. Clients are able to access health-related podcasts to acquire information about a variety of topics [51]. Through an online website called Anxiety and Depression Association of America, one can find a wide variety of podcasts on disorders ranging from social anxiety to depression in youth [52].

Online-based psychoeducation allows users to tailor pace and volume of information at their own convenience. Computer technology also has the ability to appear unbiased and unassociated with control and authority, which are often identified with educators [53]. An example of a computer intervention is MoodGYM, an anxiety and depression website that provides youth with informational resources, thereby improving client's overall attitudes and knowledge without the presence of parents or other perceived stressors [54]. It is important that therapists using CIT for psychoeducation purposes identify specific and reliable resources to suggest for their clients. There exists significant misinformation online, and before offering psychoeducative resources, a therapist should evaluate the accuracy of such a resource.

The following is an example of ways to use CIT for psychoeducation:

Case Study

Juan is a 12-year-old Latino male who immigrated to Los Angeles, California, with his family a year ago. Despite being a social child back in Mexico, Juan is struggling with leaving his house and the care of his parents. He refuses to go to school by himself and is afraid he will never see his family again if he is separated from them. In Mexico, Juan lived with many of his extended family members as well as another family, totaling 20 in the household. He would often be very social at school and on the playground and was seen as a "social butterfly." At school in Mexico, Juan was at the top of his class when it came to typing on the computer and using the technology provided at school to find answers for his homework. Juan oftentimes finds it difficult to "fit in" and immerse himself in the games and conversations of his classmates.

Juan's therapist used multiple examples of CIT in psychoeducating Juan and his family on his current difficulties and options for treatment. Juan showed an interest in using new and upcoming technology at school and at home. He showed engagement when on a smartphone playing a game on an application, so this was the best option for Juan to partake in psychoeducation and fully understand his symptoms and possible treatment options. MoodGYM helped his therapist explain the differences between experiencing helpful and unhelpful anxiety. Using this program, the therapist also showed Juan how anxiety and habituation works to help him "fit in" and feel more connected with his peers.

During a therapy session, Juan's therapist used different CIT options such as a smartphone application or an Internet intervention to understand why he is experiencing these symptoms. It was important for Juan and his therapist to discuss how and why the client may be experiencing social anxiety along with the thoughts and behaviors behind it. It was important to use technology and information for psychoeducation that was easy for Juan to understand and to tailor the therapy for each specific client. Also, Juan was not an English speaker, and the therapist had to take into consideration language abilities and different CIT psychoeducation options in his native language so that Juan and his family could clearly understand his symptoms, causes, and treatments available for his social anxiety.

Technology and Relaxation Strategies

Relaxation training (RT) has been found to be an effective method for reducing psychological problems in youth [55]. Stress and anxiety reduction and improved self-esteem and self-concept are just a few of the benefits of RT. More recently, innovative forms of RT have been created to engage youth through the use of technology [3]. From videogames to phone apps, technology-enhanced relaxation techniques can be used to treat anxiety-related issues in immigrant youth. For example, a number of studies have found that playing classical music and nature sounds for even just a small amount of time, such as in 5-min intervals, significantly reduces heart rate and blood pressure associated with mental stress [56–58]. Similar to applications that play relaxing music are audio CDs designed for relaxation. According to Chu et al. [45], relaxation CDs can effectively reduce anxiety in youth due to motivational increases and the ability to be played outside of session repeatedly. Another advantage is that CDs do not require the presence of a therapist and can be used for practicing when the client is at home.

The following is an example of ways to use CIT for relaxation training:

Case Study

Imelda is a 13-year-old Filipino female who immigrated to Southern California approximately 6 months ago. She currently lives with her aunt, uncle, and two cousins; they have been US residents for a decade. In school, Imelda is academically strong but suffers socially. She has low self-esteem which prevents her from reaching out to others and making friends. Additionally, Imelda's high levels of anxiety make it difficult to hold conversations with peers. Therapists can use several technology-based relaxation techniques to address Imelda's problems.

Imelda and her therapist used Internet radio apps to find a number of relaxing stations for her to use when feeling stressed. Another similar app they used was "Feel Good" which is specifically designed as a relaxing break from a daily routine. This application used music coupled with relaxing imagery to induce calmness. Introducing Imelda to relaxation apps and instructing her on their use helped to ease some cognitive and physical symptoms associated with her anxiety.

Audio CDs were a good option for Imelda because she practiced regulating her anxiety independently at home and transferred that knowledge to her school setting.

A less conventional form of technology that used for RT with Imelda were video games. Currently there are a number of biofeedback video games that train youth to recognize and manipulate their body's physiological responses to anxiety and stress. Imelda played The Journey to Wild Divine, which taught her breathing skills and muscle relaxation by measuring heart rate and skin conductance levels, resulting in significant reductions in anxiety symptoms. This technology was useful in training Imelda to overcome her anxiety symptoms when in social situations, thus improving her self-concept and social skills.

Incorporating technology into relaxation techniques with youth has been shown to be an effective form of alleviating anxiety, stress, and self-esteem problems. However, relaxation is a term that is strongly tied to culture. For example, a study by Yeh and Inose [24] found that Korean immigrant youths are more likely to seek religious services as a method of coping as compared to other immigrants of East Asian descent. An important aspect for therapists to consider when working with immigrant youth is finding a culturally appropriate way of employing technology.

Cognitive Restructuring

Cognitive restructuring helps to reduce negative provoking "self-talk" and helps youth build stronger coping strategies [59, p. 122]. Therapists challenge negative thinking by questioning the evidence behind these thoughts, challenging erroneous beliefs, using repeated exposure to feared situations [60], and continuously engaging youth in the process [59]. The use of the Internet may assist psychotherapists to challenge an immigrant youth's maladaptive thinking, especially with misconception of ideas and beliefs, by providing an effective way to find information, data, and resources regarding their beliefs.

The following is an example of ways to use CIT for cognitive restructuring:

Case Study

Aadita is a 17-year-old female from Jaipur, India, who moved to New York with her family a year ago. She has been experiencing anxiety symptoms that began a month ago after watching a new popular zombie movie. Her symptoms have progressively worsened, interfere with her ability to do her school work, and caused her to miss a month of school. Aadita fears that zombies are going to attack her and her family, especially during the night when she goes to sleep. She knows these fears are irrational, but she cannot help feeling nervous and tense; she keeps imagining the grotesque zombies will eat her.

By using the Internet, her therapist helped Aadita to challenge her maladaptive thoughts. Aadita searched for online images and videos of zombie makeup transformation. The Internet provided many documentaries about the making of zombie movies and the hours of training on how to behave like a zombie. Aadita and her therapist also created their own avatar zombies using a website/smartphone application called ZombieMe.com: a free program that creates a monster or zombie using an image of your own face. By learning of the story behind developing monster movies and the effects employed by the zombie movie, Aadita helped recognize the people behind the makeup and visual effects that terrified her.

Additionally, the therapist worked together with Aadita in setting reminders on her mobile phone with questions to challenge her thoughts. Questions included: Is thinking about zombies helpful? Are my thoughts about zombies realistic? What evidence is there for and against the existence of zombies? What did I learn about zombies that that makes me feel better? What can I say to myself that will help me remain calm?

CIT for Exposure

Engagement in hierarchy-based exposure tasks is often considered the most important component of the treatment of anxiety disorders [61, 62]. During treatment with exposure, youths face their fears while developing adaptive behavior in response to a feared stimulus or situation [63]. CIT has the ability to effectively treat anxiety and phobia disorders through exposure exercises.

Using the Internet to deliver cognitive behavioral therapy interventions has been found to be effective in the treatment of children with specific phobia [9]. With adult populations, Internet-based exposure therapies have been found to reduce symptoms related to several anxiety disorders and obsessive-compulsive disorder [64–68]. Internet studies have found effects maintained over time, especially in participants that have access to treatment material after the study has ended [69]. Additionally, Andersson and colleagues [66] found that Internet-guided exposure can be accomplished without meeting face-to-face using four Internet and video modules that present methods for finding and interacting with feared stimuli in graduated levels of exposure.

Migration stressors have shown to increase the risk for both depressive and anxiety symptoms [70]. For example, Latino immigrant adolescents in families with undocumented members, where identification could have consequences including arrest or deportation, are at higher risk of anxiety [70, 71]. In these cases, treatment using the Internet or other distanced communication technologies could be an alternative to traditional face-to-face therapy in order to lessen immigrant status anxiety. However, care should be taken to avoid overexposure when away from the relative safety of the therapist's presence.

The following is an example of ways to use CIT for exposure:

Case Study

Sofia is a 14-year-old Haitian girl who moved to Massachusetts to live with her father, who is an undocumented immigrant. She recently told the school counselor that she has been unable to meet with friends who live in wooded areas, indicating symptoms of specific phobia to bears, which are not native to Haiti. She admits that therapy would be helpful for her, but is hesitant due to her father's immigration status.

In Sofia's case, her therapist used Internet modules which begin with pictures of bears, before moving to videos, and eventually a visit to a zoo or guided wildlife refuge tours to interact with real bears in safe situations. These Internet-guided exposure modules were effective in reducing Sofia's anxiety symptoms. In addition, conducting her exposure therapy via the Internet allowed Sofia to distance herself from the therapist, thereby alleviating her worries surrounding her father's immigration status.

Virtual reality is another way that exposure therapy can help clients deal with the anxiety of unknown stimuli and situations. Virtual reality exposure (VRE) used for anxiety and phobias allows clients to control the level of exposure without sacrificing the alliance with their therapist. VRE assists clinicians with motivation and provides the same support and problem-solving coping skills as traditional in vivo or imagined exposure procedures. There is limited research with youth, but VRE has shown to be just as effective in treatment outcome as with adults in traditional exposure interventions [45]. The barriers to use for virtual reality have drastically lowered in recent years, such as cardboard headsets that can be placed over a smartphone screen, increasing the viability of VRE as a therapeutic intervention.

Relapse Prevention

A critical component of psychological intervention is the maintenance of therapeutic gains or relapse prevention (RP). The main objective of RP is to facilitate lifestyle changes that will reduce the risk of future psychological stress by reinforcing the achieved goals and consolidating what has been learned [72]. CIT can help clients to retain learned skills and achievements by creating fun and engaging stories, advertisements, movies, and drawings [73].

The following is an example of ways to use CIT for relapse prevention:

Case Study

Carlos is a 10-year-old Mexican boy who migrated from Jalisco to Los Angeles (LA) approximately 1 year ago. Carlos lives with his mother and three sisters in a small apartment in East LA. He exhibited frequent angry outbursts both at school and home. Carlos had social integration difficulties and on several occasions initiated physical fights related to antiforeigner sentiment. After working with a psychotherapist, Carlos has increased his social and anger management skills. Now, in the final sessions of therapy, there are several techniques that Carlos can use to maintain his new skills.

A study by Rooney et al. [74] found that youth can improve attentional skills through self-recording, thereby increasing the ability to learn and maintain new skills. Instructing Carlos to enact and describe specific treatment models will reinforce his newly acquired skills and serve as a reference should he forget was learned in therapy. Furthermore, video recording will provide Carlos with an engrossing learning activity that promotes pride. Carlos' recording can act as a "trophy" that visually illustrates his accomplishments in therapy [75].

Carlos can also maintain therapeutic solutions through the utilization of visual aids which are an effective form of improving decision-making and reducing unwanted behaviors [43]. With the therapist, Carlos can create a flowchart where he can identify trigger scenarios and identify the appropriate coping skills learned in therapy. The flowchart provides Carlos access to reactive strategies that can maintain newly acquired skills and reduce relapse rates. Computer programs and online chart generators easily create clear and concise "roadmaps" that Carlos can use to successfully interact outside of therapy. Incorporating a computer will keep Carlos engaged in the task while simultaneously providing him with a tool for learning.

Although often overlooked, RP is an important part of any intervention. RP prepares the client for situations that he or she may face when no longer in session [59]. Integrating CIT is a useful resource in reinforcing therapeutic gains and fostering ongoing learning. Additionally, the use of technology is an interactive way to engage immigrant youth in tasks that may otherwise seem mundane.

Telepsychotherapy

Telepsychotherapy is the use of electronic media, telephone (landlines or cellular), and videoconferencing as a means of delivering psychotherapeutic services [6]. Telepsychotherapy provides a psychotherapist and immigrant youth a way to conduct therapeutic sessions from different locations when access to healthcare providers is limited because of remote geographical locations or lack of public transportation [76, 77]. Immigrant youth may also benefit from telepsychotherapy by minimizing time and travel expenses [78, 79]. For example, they could contact therapists still residing in their home country or culture. In particular, youth are more likely to engage via video conferencing, thereby reducing anxiety and barriers to treatment [78, 79]. Although telepsychotherapy may be a convenient modality for immigrant youth when in-person sessions are not feasible, there are also several risks involved (see section "Ethical Considerations").

Digital Psychotherapy

Digital psychotherapy is designed to enhance therapist-client sessions using various forms of technology such as computer programs, smartphone apps, or online interventions (previously defined as Computer Assisted Psychotherapy—Write, 2008; for a review, see Cucciare and Weingardt [80]). This type of psychotherapy can be tailored for each specific client based on severity of disorder and necessity of face-to-face contact with clinicians [81] while still allowing client and therapist to meet, build a therapeutic relationship, and discuss difficult issues that a client may tend to avoid when using a computer program [81]. An example of this is a CD-ROM called Camp Cope-A-Lot for treating anxiety disorders in youth [82]. This program incorporates video game levels and kid-friendly graphics to promote interactive participation and simplistic maintenance and reduction of symptoms and negative coping mechanisms. This digital program in complement to face-to-face psychotherapy has been found to be effective in the reduction of anxiety and increased overall functioning [82]. As the main character of the program is a cat, this may allow youth of diverse ethnic backgrounds to identify with it.

Digital Self-Help

Digital self-help interventions are treatments operationalized and adapted for Web or mobile device delivery without the presence of the therapist (Adapted from Muñoz [42]). Although no digital self-help interventions have been tested with immigrant youth, they may be useful and effective in reducing and preventing disorders such as depression and anxiety. Two examples of such programs are CATCH-IT and BRAVE. CATCH-IT is a preventative Internet-based intervention that targets depression in adolescents using 14 CBT modules, which are designed to increase motivation by decreasing maladaptive behaviors [83]. BRAVE is a CBT-based program for youth with anxiety disorders delivered entirely via the Internet and is effective in reducing anxiety symptoms in adolescents [84]. For a review on digital self-help interventions, see Richardson et al. [85].

Digital psychotherapy and digital self-help interventions are easy to access at the convenience of immigrant youth, who may not have the finances or transportation to visit and pay for a therapist [81]. Also, digital interventions reduce the stigma of seeing a traditional therapist and can be done in privacy of their own home [84]. As such, these evidence-based digital interventions may be a viable option for psychological treatment of disorders in immigrant youth.

Ethical Considerations

Several ethical considerations must be addressed as the field of psychotherapy moves towards CIT utilization. The American Psychological Association issued a comprehensive report in July 2013 elaborating ethical guidelines for conducting telepsychotherapy which include competency with associated technologies (e.g., computers, mobile phones, etc.), confidentiality of information, electronic privacy, and informed consent (APA [86]). The APA states that psychologists seeking to communicate via the Internet or phone calls must understand the risks and benefits of the related communication method. For example, Internet and mobile phone communication can allow for interaction over long distances, but therapists must be wary of potential Internet outages or dropped calls. The APA also warns that therapists need to be aware of encryption and data security, highlighting that confidentiality and privacy on the Internet and in phone calls cannot be guaranteed. Clients need to be aware of these risks to telepsychotherapy and the information must be included in informed consent [86].

The Division 29 Task Force, responsible for the advancement of psychotherapy, recommends that, as a first step, psychotherapists should check with their state laws regarding the regulations of telepsychotherapy. Also, should the client reside in a different state, the psychotherapist must check with the state licensing board to make sure both states approve the use of telepsychotherapy. Another major concern is the decrease in the psychotherapist's control over the environmental settings, interpersonal dynamics, and building rapport [78, 79]. Similar to other therapeutic modalities, challenges of working with immigrant youth using telepsychotherapy include cultural differences, language barriers, prejudice, preparing therapists to accommodate differences, efficacy, and effectiveness versus the costs [79, 87]. There are many skeptics to the idea of therapy through the use of telecommunication. Deen and colleagues [76] mention that telepsychotherapy is a better option than a potential client receiving no health services. It is important that clients are properly informed of their rights and limits to confidentiality when under the care of a psychotherapist who practices telepsychotherapy.

Conclusions

Immigrant youth may face a wide spectrum of physical and psychological barriers as they transition to their new host country and cultural surroundings. CIT may be beneficial for immigrant youth by providing resources for health-related services to promote cultural, social, physical, and psychological adaptation [34, 88]. There are four ways that CIT may help in adaptation: through utilizing social media, by enhancing face-to-face psychotherapy/telepsychotherapy, including digital interventions into psychotherapy, and providing digital self-help resources. Social media may enhance the adjustment to the new culture and provide a social connection between the immigrant youth and those he or she left behind [29]. CIT may help in every phase of face-to-face psychotherapy, customizing interactions with digitally native immigrant youth [29, 66, 89, 90]. In digital psychotherapy, there is therapist involvement in digital interventions such as captivating computer programs and smartphone apps [90]. Digital self-help treatment is operationalized in adapted Web and mobile applications without therapist involvement [84]. Finally, CIT is a constantly evolving field, which can help break down migration barriers and provide generationally adaptive mental health resources for immigrant youth.

References

1. Friedberg RD, Hoyman LC, Behar S, Tabbarah S, Pacholec NM, Keller M, Thordarson MA. We've come a long way, baby!: Evolution and revolution in CBT with youth. J Ration Emot Cogn Behav Ther. 2014;32(1):4–14.
2. Thinyane H. Are digital natives a world-wide phenomenon? An investigation into South African first year students' use and experience with technology. Comput Educ. 2010; 55(1):406–14.
3. Amon KL, Campbell A. Can Children with AD/HD learn relaxation and breathing techniques through biofeedback video games? Aust J Educ Dev Psychol. 2008;8(1):72–84.
4. Ceranoglu TA. Video games in psychotherapy. Rev Gen Psychol. 2010;14(2):141–6. doi:10.1037/a0019439.

5. Dingfelder SF. Giving psychology away, one podcast at a time. Monitor on Psychology. 2010;41:31. Retrieved from http://www.apa.org/monitor/2010/02/podcast.aspx

6. Judge AB, Abeles N, Davis SP, Adam-Terem R, Younggren JN. Report from the task force on telepsychotherapy. American Psychological Association, Division 29; 2011. Retrieved Oct 1, 2014 from http://www.divisionofpsychotherapy.org/report-from-the-task-force-on-telepsychotherapy/

7. Kato PM. Video games in health care: closing the gap. Rev Gen Psychol. 2010;14(2):113–21. doi:10.1037/a0019441.

8. Luxton DD, McCann RA, Bush NE, Mishkind MC, Reger GM. mHealth for mental health: Integrating smartphone technology in behavioral healthcare. Prof Psychol Res Pract. 2011;42(6):505.

9. Vigerland S, Thulin U, Ljótsson B, Svirsky L, Öst LG, Lindefors N, et al. Internet-delivered CBT for children with specific phobia: a pilot study. Cogn Behav Ther. 2013;42(4):303–14. doi:10.1080/16506073.2013.844201.

10. Norcross JC, Pfund RA, Prochaska JO. Psychotherapy in 2022: a Delphi poll on its future. Prof Psychol Res Pract. 2013;44(5):363–70. doi:10.1037/a0034633.

11. Zur O, Zur A. On digital immigrants and digital natives: how the digital divide affects families, educational institutions, and the workplace. Zur Institute - Innovative Resources & Online Continuing Education; 2011. Retrieved from http://www.zurinstitute.com/digital_divide.html

12. Sallai G. Defining infocommunications and related terms. Acta Polytechnica Hungarica. 2012;9(6):5–15.

13. Pearce KE, Rice RE. Digital divides from access to activities: comparing mobile and personal computer internet users. J Commun. 2013;63(4):721–44.

14. Hoffman DL, Novak TP. Bridging the racial divide on the internet: the impact of race on computer access and internet use. Science. 1998;280(5362):390–1.

15. Kind T, Huang ZJ, Farr D, Pomerantz KL. Internet and computer access and use for health information in an underserved community. Ambul Pediatr. 2005;5(2):117–21.

16. van Dijk, JA. A theory of the digital divide 1. The Digital Divide. 2013;29.

17. Howard PN, Busch L, Sheets P. Comparing digital divides: internet access and social inequality in Canada and the United States. Can J Commun. 2010;35:109–28.

18. Ono H, Zavodny M. Immigrants, English ability and the digital divide. Soc Forces. 2008;86(4):1455–79.

19. Van Deursen A, Van Dijk J. The digital divide shifts to differences in usage. New Media Soc. 2014;16(3):507–26. doi:10.1177/1461444813487959.

20. Bertot JC, Jaeger PT, Langa LA, McClure CR. Public access computing and Internet access in public libraries: the role of public libraries in e-government and emergency situations. First Monday. 2006;11(9). doi:10.5210/fm.v11i9.139

21. Jaeger PT, Bertot JC, McClure CR, Rodriguez M. Public libraries and Internet access across the United States: a comparison by state 2004–2006. Inf Technol Libr. 2013;26(2):4–14.

22. James D. Coping with a new society: the unique psychosocial problems of immigrant youth. J Sch Health. 1997;67(3):98–102.

23. Yeh C. Age, acculturation, cultural adjustment, and mental health symptoms of Chinese, Korean, and Japanese immigrant youths. Cult Divers Ethn Minor Psychol. 2003;9(1):34–48. doi:10.1037/10999809.9.1.34.

24. Yeh C, Inose M. Difficulties and coping strategies of Chinese, Japanese and Korean immigrant students. Adolescence. 2002;37(145):69–82.

25. Mirsky J. Mental health implications of migration. Soc Psychiatry Psychiatr Epidemiol. 2009;44(3):179–87.

26. Buckingham D, De Block L. Finding a global voice? Migrant children, new media and the limits of empowerment. In: Dahlgren P, editor. Young citizens and new media: learning for democratic participation. Routledge: Abingdon; 2007. p. 147–63.

27. Elias N, Lemish D. Media uses in immigrant families: torn between 'inward' and 'outward' paths of integration. Int Commun Gaz. 2008;70(1):21–40. doi:10.1177/1748048507084576.

28. Zohoori AR. A cross-cultural analysis of children's television use. J Broadcast Electron Media. 1988;32(1):105–13. doi:10.1080/08838158809386687.

29. Elias N, Lemish D. Spinning the web of identity: the roles of the internet in the lives of immigrant adolescents. New Media Soc. 2009;11(4):533–51. doi:10.1177/1461444809102959.

30. Livingstone S, Bober M. Taking up online opportunities? Children's uses of the internet for education, communication and participation. E-Learning. 2004;1(3):395–419.

31. Mesch GS, Talmud I. Similarity and the quality of online and offline social relationships among adolescents in Israel. J Res Adolesc. 2007;17(2):455–65.

32. Valentine G, Holloway SL. Cyberkids? Exploring children's identities and social networks in online and offline worlds. Ann Assoc Am Geogr. 2002;92(2):302–19.

33. Valkenburg PM, Peter J. Preadolescents' and adolescents' online communication and their closeness to friends. Dev Psychol. 2007;43(2):267–77. doi:10.1037/0012-1649.43.2.267.

34. Rhodes J. Research corner: mentoring immigrant youth. Mentor National Mentoring Partnership; 2005. Retrieved from http://www.mentoring.or/downloads/mentoring_1318.pdf

35. Gonzales AL, Hancock JT. Mirror, mirror on my Facebook wall: effects of exposure to Facebook on self-esteem. Cyberpsychol Behav Soc Netw. 2011;14(1-2):79–83. doi:10.1089/cyber.2009.0411.

36. Lee SY. How do people compare themselves with others on social network sites?: The case of facebook. Comput Hum Behav. 2014;32:253–60.

37. Facebook. Company info. Facebook Newsroom; 2014. Retrieved November 11, 2014, from http://newsroom.fb.com/company-info/

38. Suval L. Facebook, happiness and self-esteem; 2012. Retrieved October 1, 2014, from http://psychcentral.com/blog/archives/2012/10/04/facebook-happiness-and-self-esteem/

39. Choi M, Toma CL. Social sharing through interpersonal media: patterns and effects on emotional well-being. Comput Hum Behav. 2014;36:530–41. doi:10.1016/j.chb.2014.04.026.

40. Mitchell MA, Schmidt NB. An experimental manipulation of social comparison in social anxiety. Cogn Behav Ther. 2014;43(3):221–9. doi:10.1080/16506073.2014.914078.

41. Belfer ML. Child and adolescent mental disorders: the magnitude of the problem across the globe. J Child Psychol Psychiatry. 2008;49(3):226–36. doi:10.1111/j.1469-7610.2007.01855.x.

42. Muñoz RF. Using evidence-based internet interventions to reduce health disparities worldwide. J Med Internet Res. 2010;12(5).

43. Garcia-Retamero R, Cokely ET. Communicating health risks with visual aids. Curr Dir Psychol Sci. 2013;22(5):392–9. doi:10.1177/0963721413491570.

44. Kazdin AE, Blase SL. Rebooting psychotherapy research and practice to reduce the burden of mental illness. Perspect Psychol Sci. 2011;6(1):21–37. doi:10.1177/1745691610393527.

45. Chu BC, Choudhury MS, Shortt AL, Pincus DB, Creed TA, Kendall PC. Alliance, technology, and outcome in the treatment of anxious youth. Cogn Behav Pract. 2004;11(1):44–55. doi:10.1016/S1077-7229(04)80006-3.

46. Boschen MJ, Casey LM. The use of mobile telephones as adjuncts to cognitive behavioral psychotherapy. Prof Psychol Res Pr. 2008;39(5):546. doi:10.1037/0735-7028.39.5.546.

47. Brown JR, Holloway ED, Akakpo TF, Aalsma MC. "Straight up": enhancing rapport and therapeutic alliance with previously-detained youth in the delivery of mental health services. Community Ment Health J. 2014;50(2):193–203. doi:10.1007/s10597-013-9617-3.

48. Brezinka V. Computer games supporting cognitive behaviour therapy in children. Clin Child Psychol Psychiatry. 2014;19(1):100–10. doi:10.1177/1359104512468288.

49. Elliott D. Levelling the playing field: engaging disadvantaged students through game-based pedagogy. Lit Learn Middle Years. 2014;22(2):34–40.

50. Rotondi A, Anderson C, Haas G, Eack S, Spring M, Ganguli R, et al. Web-based psychoeducational intervention for persons with schizophrenia and their supporters: one-year outcomes. Psychiatr Serv. 2010;61(11):1099–105. doi:10.1176/appi.ps.61.11.1099.

51. Boulos MN, Maramba I, Wheeler S. Wikis, blogs and podcasts: a new generation of web-based tools for virtual collaborative clinical practice and education. BMC Med Educ. 2006;6(1):41–9. doi:10.1186/1472-6920-6-41.

52. Anxiety and Depression Association of American (2010, January 1). Retrieved August 26, 2014, from http://www.adaa.org/podcasts-multimedia

53. Andrewes DG, Mulder C, O'connor P, McLennan J, Say S, Derham H, Weigall S. Computerised psychoeducation for patients with eating disorders. Aust N Z J Psychiatry. 1996;30(4):492–7. doi:10.3109/00048679609065022.

54. O'Kearney R, Gibson M, Christensen H, Griffiths KM. Effects of a cognitive-behavioural internet program on depression, vulnerability to depression and stigma in adolescent males: a school-based controlled trial. Cogn Behav Ther. 2006;35(1):43–54. doi:10.1080/16506070500303456.

55. Lohaus A, Klein-Hessling J. Relaxation in children: effects of extended and intensified training. Psychol Health. 2003;18(2):237–49. doi:10.1080/0887044021000057257.

56. Robb SL. The effect of therapeutic music interventions on the behavior of hospitalized children in isolation: developing a contextual support model of music therapy. J Music Ther. 2000;37(2):118–46.

57. Scheufele PM. Effects of progressive relaxation and classical music on measurements of attention, relaxation, and stress responses. J Behav Med. 2000;23(2):207–28.

58. Sung BH, Roussanov O, Nagubandi M, Golden L. A002: Effectiveness of various relaxation techniques in lowering blood pressure associated with mental stress. Am J Hypertens. 2000;13(S2):185A.

59. Friedberg RD, McClure JM, Garcia JH. Cognitive therapy techniques for children and adolescents: tools for enhancing practice. New York, NY: Guilford; 2009.

60. Castonguay LG, Beutler LE, editors. Principles of therapeutic change that work. New York: Oxford University Press; 2006.

61. Bouchard S, Mendlowitz SL, Coles ME, Franklin M. Considerations in the use of exposure with children. Cogn Behav Pract. 2004;11(1):56–65. doi:10.1016/S1077-7229(04)80007-5.

62. Kendall PC, Robin JA, Hedtke KA, Gosch E, Flannery-Schroeder E, Suveg C. Conducting CBT with anxious youth? Think exposures. Cogn Behav Pract. 2005;12(1):136–50. doi:10.1016/S1077-7229(05)80048-3.

63. Benjamin CL, Podell JL, Mychailyszyn MP, Puleo CM, Tiwari S, Kendall PC. Cognitive-behavioral therapy for child anxiety: key components. In: Gomar M, Mandil J, Bunge E, editors. Handbook of cognitive behavioral therapy with children and adolescents. Buenos Aires: Polemos; 2010. p. 207–40.

64. Andersson E, Enander J, Andrén P, Hedman E, Ljótsson B, Hursti T, et al. Internet-based cognitive behaviour therapy for obsessive-compulsive disorder: a randomized controlled trial. Psychol Med. 2012;42(10):2193–203. doi:10.1017/S0033291712000244.

65. Andersson G, Carlbring P, Holmström A, Sparthan E, Furmark T, Nilsson-Ihrfelt E, et al. Internet-based self-help with therapist feedback and in vivo group exposure for social phobia: a randomized controlled trial. J Consult Clin Psychol. 2006;74(4):677–86. doi: 10.1037/0022-006X.74.4.677.

66. Andersson G, Waara J, Jonsson U, Malmaeus F, Carlbring P, Ost L-G. Internet-based exposure treatment versus one-session exposure treatment of snake phobia: a randomized controlled trial. Cogn Behav Ther. 2013;42(4):284–91. doi:10.1080/16506073.2013.844202.

67. Hedman E, Andersson G, Andersson E, Ljótsson B, Rück C, Asmundson G, Lindefors N. Internet-based cognitive-behavioral therapy for severe health anxiety: randomised controlled trial. Br J Psychiatry. 2011;198(3):230–6. doi:10.1192/bjp.bp.110.086843.

68. Paxling B, Lundgren S, Norman A, Almlöv J, Carlbring P, Cuijpers P, Andersson G. Therapist behaviours in internet-delivered cognitive behaviour therapy: analysis of e-mail correspondence in the treatment of generalized anxiety disorder. Behav Cogn Psychother. 2013;41:280–9. doi:10.1017/S1352465812000240.

69. Carlbring P, Bergman L, Nordgren LB, Furmark T, Andersson G. Long-term outcome of internet-delivered cognitive–behavioural therapy for social phobia: a 30-month follow-up. Behav Res Ther. 2009;47(10):848–50. doi:10.1016/j.brat.2009.06.012.

70. Potochnick S, Perreira K. Depression and anxiety among first-generation immigrant Latino youth: key correlates and implications for future research. J Nerv Ment Dis. 2010;198(7):470–7. doi:10.1097/NMD.0b013e3181e4ce24.

71. Arbona C, Olvera N, Rodriguez N, Hagan J, Linares A, Wiesner M. Acculturative stress among documented and undocumented Latino immigrants in the United States. Hisp J Behav Sci. 2010;32(3):362–84. doi:10.1177/0739986310373210.

72. Bunge E, Gomar M, Mandil J, Consoli A. Clinical resources for cognitive behavioral therapy with anxious and depressed children and adolescents. Manuscript submitted for publication.

73. Asarnow JR, Scott CV, Mintz J. A combined cognitive–behavioral family education intervention for depression in children: a treatment development study. Cogn Ther Res. 2002;26(2): 221–9.

74. Rooney KJ, Hallahan DP, Lloyd JW. Self-recording of attention by learning disabled students in the regular classroom. J Learn Disabil. 1984;17(6):360–4. doi:10.1177/002221948401700610.

75. Kaslow NJ, Broth MR, Smith CO, Collins MH. Family-based interventions for child and adolescent disorders. J Marital Fam Ther. 2012;38(1):82–100.

76. Deen T, Fortney J, Schroeder G. Patient acceptance of and initiation and engagement in telepsychotherapy in primary care. Psychiatr Serv. 2013;64(4):380–4.

77. Walton A. What students need to know about telepsychology. gradPSYCH Magazine; 2013. Retrieved October 1, 2014, from http://www.apa.org/gradpsych/2013/09/telepsychology.aspx

78. Miller TW. Telehealth issues in consulting psychology practice. Consult Psychol J Pract Res. 2006;58:82–91.

79. Rabasca L. Taking telehealth to the next step. Monitor on Psychology; 2000. Retrieved October 1, 2014, from http://www.apa.org/monitor/apr00/telehealth.aspx

80. Cucciare MA, Weingardt KR, editors. Using technology to support evidence-based behavioral health practices: a clinician's guide. New York, NY: Routledge; 2009.

81. Marks IM, Cavanagh K, Gega L. Computer-aided psychotherapy: revolution or bubble? Br J Psychiatry. 2007;191(6):471–3. doi:10.1192/bjp.bp.107.041152.

82. Khanna MS, Kendall PC. Computer-assisted CBT for child anxiety: the coping cat CD-ROM. Cogn Behav Pract. 2008;15(2):159–65. doi:10.1016/j.cbpra.2008.02.002.

83. Van Voorhees BW, Fogel J, Pomper BE, Marko M, Reid N, Watson N, et al. Adolescent dose and ratings of an internet-based depression prevention program: a randomized trial of primary care physician brief advice versus a motivational interview. J Cogn Behav Psychother. 2009;9(1):1–19.

84. Spence SH, Donovan CL, March S, Gamble A, Anderson R, Prosser S, Kenardy J. Online CBT in the treatment of child and adolescent anxiety disorders: issues in the development of BRAVE–ONLINE and two case illustrations. Behav Cogn Psychother. 2008;36(04):411–30. doi:10.1017/S135246580800444X.

85. Richardson T, Stallard P, Velleman S. Computerised cognitive behavioural therapy for the prevention and treatment of depression and anxiety in children and adolescents: a systematic review. Clin Child Family Psychol Rev. 2010;13(3):275–90. doi:10.1007/s10567-010-0069-9.

86. Legal & Regulatory Affairs Staff. APA adopts new telepsychology guidelines. Practice Central; 2013. Retrieved October 1, 2014, from http://www.apapracticecentral.org/update/2013/09-12/telepsychology-guidelines.aspx

87. Benson E. Telehealth gets back to basics. Monitor on Psychology; 2003. Retrieved June 2, 2015, from http://www.apa.org/monitor/jun03/telehealth.aspx

88. Chen W. Internet-usage patterns of immigrants in the process of intercultural adaptation. Cyberpsychol Behav Soc Netw. 2010;13(4):387–99.

89. Barrett MS, Gershkovich M. Computers and psychotherapy: are we out of a job. Psychotherapy. 2014;51(2):220–3.

90. Kendall PC, Khanna MS, Edson A, Cummings C, Sue Harris M. Computers and psychosocial treatment for child anxiety: recent advances and ongoing efforts. Depress Anxiety. 2011; 28:58–66.

Part IV

Special Circumstances for Psychotherapy for Immigrant Youth

Treating Forcibly Displaced Young People: Global Challenges in Mental Healthcare

Ruth V. Reed, Rebecca Tyrer, and Mina Fazel

Abstract

In this chapter we focus on the treatment needs of forcibly displaced children and young people. Forcibly displaced children are heterogeneous in regard to their premigration histories, their journeys to resettlement countries, and the experiences they face after arrival in a host country. Such children come from a diverse range of cultural backgrounds, and these factors in concert with current resettlement stressors create a number of challenges in identifying and implementing effective interventions and care pathways. Many forcibly displaced children do not cross international borders and face different circumstances. This chapter will highlight key features and challenges of various service delivery models in both low- and high-income settings for internally displaced children and those seeking asylum in a host country and consider how resource differences influence provision and sustainability. Case examples illustrating some of these models of interventions will be presented.

Keywords

Intervention • Multimodal • Services • Migrant • Refugee • Asylum seeker

R.V. Reed (✉) • R. Tyrer
Oxford Health NHS Foundation Trust, Warneford Hospital, Oxford, UK
e-mail: ruth.reed@psych.ox.ac.uk

M. Fazel, M.R.C.Psych., D.M.
Department of Psychiatry, University of Oxford, Warneford Hospital, Oxford OX3 7JX, UK
e-mail: mina.fazel@psych.ox.ac.uk

© Springer International Publishing Switzerland 2016
S.G. Patel, D. Reicherter (eds.), *Psychotherapy for Immigrant Youth*,
DOI 10.1007/978-3-319-24693-2_8

Introduction

It is vital to respect and harness the resilience and resourcefulness of forcibly displaced young people and their families and recognize that ultimately adaptation and positive mental health, rather than psychological difficulty, are the normative outcomes [1]. The evidence base for forcibly displaced children, especially those outside the high-income context, is limited, both with regard to reliable prevalence estimates for psychological difficulty [2, 3] and most particularly with regard to effective mental health treatments.

The global burden of forced displacement falls most heavily on the countries least equipped to provide for refugees' needs. Failed asylum seekers, undocumented migrants, unaccompanied young people, and the internally displaced are particularly vulnerable populations, who often live in areas with poor mental health provision, and if services do exist, their needs are often poorly met, if they are able to access services at all [4, 5]. There is no "ideal" model of service delivery, given the different contexts across the globe in conjunction with a rapidly fluctuating refugee population with exposures to different potentially traumatic events. Therefore, a flexible and responsive approach in service provision and a willingness to adapt and innovate locally is essential, while also recognizing that service redesign is an intervention in itself and requires evaluation of its impact on outcomes. In high-income contexts, differences relate primarily to specialist or generalist teams and whether they are based in clinics, communities, or schools. In low-income contexts, the key challenge lies in achieving sustainable provision through building local expertise.

Legal systems in most countries create an artificial dichotomy between individuals seeking asylum and other migrants, who are commonly viewed as seeking a more favorable economic situation, rather than fleeing situations of organized violence and persecution [6]. However, the reality is far more complex, and migrants represent all hues of the spectrum, from those who have experienced multiple traumatic events on a background of longstanding adversity, to those who move through free choice from one affluent state to another [6]. For all immigrants, there are common threads of cultural and linguistic adaptation and adjusting to loss of relationships, community, social status, and the sense and place of "home."

For the purposes of this chapter, we will explore the treatment considerations of a vulnerable subgroup of the migrant population: forcibly displaced children and adolescents. Not all forcibly displaced people seek asylum, and of those who do seek asylum, relatively few are ultimately granted refugee status. Whether or not they are recognized as refugees in legal terms, from a clinician's perspective, these young people are all likely to experience similar challenges as survivors of displacement, often accompanied by witnessing disturbing events and further compounded by socioeconomic deprivation. These challenges are discussed further in chapters "Immigrant Youth Life Stressors", "Trauma and Acculturative Stress", and "Immigrant Youth and Navigating Unique Systems of Treatment." This chapter will discuss issues relevant for all forcibly displaced young people; however, the term refugee will be used throughout, regardless of legal status. Case examples are used throughout the chapter to optimize the relevance for practicing clinicians, and the key messages for practice are highlighted in the text following each case.

Resettlement in the Global Context

The year 2014 saw a continuing refugee crisis, with levels of forcible displacement reaching 59.5 million, the highest on record since comprehensive statistics on forced displacement have been gathered [7]. Low- and middle-income countries (LMIC) provided asylum to 86 % of the world's refugees, and eight out of the top ten countries receiving asylum seekers were themselves experiencing war, conflict, or gross human rights violations. Using data from the UNHCR [7] Global Trends 2014 Report, the highest refugee-generating countries were Syria, Afghanistan, and Somalia and the countries accepting the most refugees were Turkey, Pakistan, and Lebanon (see Table 1).

Refugees can experience further stressful events during their migration journeys, and these have been documented to include interpersonal violence, exploitation and sexual abuse, hunger, and exhaustion, which, compounded by displacement and loss of a familiar environment, exposes them to cumulative risks to their physical, emotional, and social development [3]. This is exacerbated for unaccompanied children who, without the important psychological buffer provided by parental figures, can be at particular risk of significant psychological difficulties [8]. The impact of such events is explored extensively in chapters "Immigrant Youth Life Stressors" and "Trauma and Acculturative Stress."

Low-income countries, which receive the highest influx of refugees, unless supported by international humanitarian organizations, rarely have the resources or the means needed to set up formal refugee camps, much less to integrate new arrivals within existing communities. As a result, many refugees live in huge overcrowded informal settlements without adequate infrastructure, schools, water, sanitation, and electricity. However, the UNHCR is beginning to recognize the need to treat camps as longer-term developments rather than informal, transient settlements. Organic development of informal camps driven by refugees is taking place, for example, at Zaatari, a refugee camp home to approximately 85,000 Syrians in Jordan, which is becoming an informal city with a growing economy [9]. Many

Table 1 Top 10 highest refugee-generating and refugee receiving countries by the end of 2014 [7]

Highest refugee-generating countries	Highest refugee-receiving countries
Syrian Arab Rep. (3.9 million)	Turkey (1.6 million)
Afghanistan (2.6 million)	Pakistan (1.5 million)
Somalia (1.11 million)	Lebanon (1.15 million)
Sudan (666,000)	Islamic Rep. of Iran (5.2 million)
South Sudan (616,200)	Ethiopia (659,500)
Dem. Rep. of the Congo (516,800)	Jordon (654,100)
Myanmar (479,000)	Kenya (551,400)
Central African Rep. (412,000)	Chad (452,900)
Iraq (369,900)	Uganda (385,500)
Eritrea (363,100)	China (301,000)

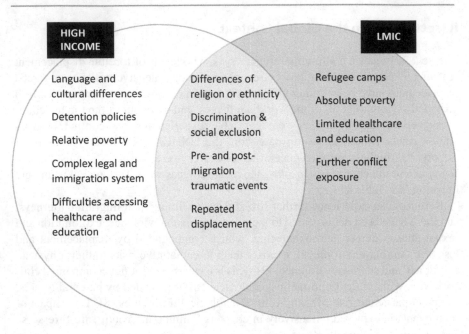

HIGH INCOME

LMIC

Language and cultural differences

Detention policies

Relative poverty

Complex legal and immigration system

Difficulties accessing healthcare and education

Differences of religion or ethnicity

Discrimination & social exclusion

Pre- and post-migration traumatic events

Repeated displacement

Refugee camps

Absolute poverty

Limited healthcare and education

Further conflict exposure

Fig. 1

refugees live in informal refugee camps without any possibility of cultivating land, seeking employment opportunities, or an education, due to state-imposed restrictions [10]. Such living conditions can contribute to psychological difficulties for the growing numbers of children who face poor health and malnutrition, limited education, parents unable or not permitted to work, and increased exposure to abuse and violence in the context of extreme family and community stress [3, 11].

Conflict not only has direct effects on mental health, but also contributes to psychological distress indirectly through cumulative daily hassles [12]. Taking these factors into consideration, Miller and Rasmussen discussed how interventions should be implemented. They suggest that the first level of intervention is at the psychosocial level, seeking to reduce daily difficulties such as violence, malnutrition, and demoralization, which will have a substantial impact on psychological distress for many affected people. Those who remain severely affected or traumatized despite such psychosocial approaches can then be identified for individually targeted psychological interventions.

The enormity of the challenges in LMIC settings should not inure us to the difficulties encountered in high-income settings, where children must learn a new language, acculturate to complex societies often alongside exposure to "anti-asylum" sentiment and social isolation [13]. Some of the vulnerabilities, and similarities or differences between HIC (high-income country) and LMIC (low- and middle-income country) contexts, are illustrated in Fig. 1, while Case 1 shows the extreme adversity faced by failed asylum seekers in the HIC context.

Case Study 1: The Situation of Failed Asylum Seekers

Marie is an 18-year-old Congolese woman who arrived in the UK as an unaccompanied asylum seeker, at the age of 15. Her asylum claim was rejected when she reached the age of 18, and she has exhausted all her rights of appeal. She has been told she must leave the host country but sleeps on her friend Emma's sofa in exchange for childcare, cooking, and cleaning. Marie is frightened that the authorities will find her. Before her appeal failed, she had received intermitted support for depression and PTSD from health services, but the uncertainty of her asylum status and place of residence had meant she had not felt ready to undertake trauma-focused psychological therapy. Emma is concerned that Marie is very low in mood, but she can no longer access the mental health clinic as she now has no rights to non-emergency care. She refuses to see a doctor in any case, for fear they will report her to the immigration authorities, so she has no further access to antidepressants. Marie accepts attending a refugee charity for confidential counseling, but does not seem any better.

The situation of those who have exhausted the appeals process in HIC but still feel unsafe or unwilling to return to their country can be particularly desperate. Not only do they live with the threat of removal and social deprivation, but they are also unable to access basic care, as illustrated in Case Example 1.

Government policies for the treatment of asylum-seeking children are fraught with difficulties, and children suffer the consequences of the declined immigration applications of their parents. For example, in the UK, if families refuse to cooperate with deportation, children may be forced to separate from their parents and taken into care by social services. The potential implications for children as a result of destitution and separation from their family has not yet been widely explored, but such policies are clearly of concern in their potential negative impact on child and adult mental health [14].

Immigrant and refugee populations have often experienced prolonged separation from key family members, with some studies reporting that up to 85 % of immigrant adolescents have experienced separation from their parents [15]. These separations can be for different reasons including financial restrictions and complex immigration policies [16]. Some children might remain with extended families, while others might be placed with unfamiliar caregivers. In 2011, as a result of parent deportation or arrest over immigration disputes in the USA, over 5000 children were placed in foster care [17], while parents were forced to return to their country of origin to apply for permanent residence, often taking months or years before being allowed to return [18]. The subsequent reunifications can be fraught with difficulties [15, 19–22]. Recent US legislation has sought to improve children's welfare by enabling applications to be submitted within the USA [18] and introducing a fast-track process for family immigration [23]. While this legislation is an important step, a substantial number of children still experience prolonged separation, not only in the

USA, but across the globe [24]. Although there is longitudinal data from non-refugee migrant young people indicating that the impact of parental separation may be a short-to medium-term rather than long-term risk factor for psychological difficulty [25], it is important to note that the reasons for parental separation and likelihood of maintaining some form of contact or achieving reunification with parents often differ between migrant and unaccompanied asylum-seeking populations. This limits the relevance of findings from existing research on non-refugee migrant populations in relation to young refugees.

Challenges

Prevalence of Mental Health Problems

The most common mental health problems among forcibly displaced young people are anxiety, depression, and a range of responses to potentially traumatic events, including PTSD [26]. Their caregivers are also at elevated risk of the same conditions, and caregiver and child mental health show an interrelationship in refugee populations as in other spheres [2]. Estimates of prevalence vary substantially depending upon the population studied. Rates are affected by prior rates of psychological difficulty and exposure to adversity, the nature and degree of previous exposure to potentially traumatic events (PTEs), and the prevailing conditions after migration, most particularly further exposure to adversity, instability, and PTEs [2, 3].

Risk and Protective Factors

The prevalence of anxiety, depression, and PTEs among young refugees is generally substantially higher than their peers in host populations, given the different balance of risk and protective factors between the two populations. These risk and protective factors were explored in paired systematic reviews, with differences across HIC and LMIC contexts highlighted [2, 3]. Child and parent exposure to premigration violence, child exposure to post-migration violence, changes of residence, perceived discrimination, being unaccompanied, and being female were identified as risk factors for poor mental health in studies in HIC [2]. Family cohesion, social support, a positive school experience, and same ethnic-origin foster care were associated with better mental health. In LMIC, exposure to premigration violence, settlement in a refugee camp rather than within a host community, and internal displacement were found to be risk factors; as in host populations, females were at elevated risk for internalizing problems and males for externalizing problems [3]. Children who left a country with active conflict and were subsequently repatriated fared better than those who remained in the conflict situation, but there is a lack of evidence on whether such children would fare better remaining in the host country than being repatriated. The latter is a complex question which requires an assessment of the balance between the disadvantages of further social, educational, and economic disruption by repatriation, versus the advantages of returning to a familiar cultural and linguistic environment; this balance may well differ depending upon length of time in the host country and the stability and conditions of the country of origin, and moreover the balance of risk and benefit may differ between parents and children, who vary in their adaptability to new environments.

Mental Health Needs Over Time

Health needs and therefore service provision may need to differ for newly arrived populations compared to longer-term resettled young people. Challenges in the provision of care for new arrivals are a high burden of distress from recent traumatic events, a lack of familiarity with the language and local systems, and the unintentionally inappropriate use of health systems to seek help with social and legal problems. Moreover, there are frequent changes in the predominant countries of origin for asylum seekers, depending on the world political situation. This can affect the availability and quality of interpreters for consultations and clinician familiarity with appropriate cultural adaptations of care. Over the long term, prolonged uncertainty and ongoing social exclusion can exert negative effects on mental health, particularly when occurring in the context of adolescent identity development.

Longitudinal studies are particularly challenging for highly mobile populations such as refugees. Those studies which have been completed indicate that the burden of psychological difficulty seems to reduce over time [27], and most young people have positive outcomes [28, 29]. Behavioral problems and substance misuse are low, and most young people successfully enter education or employment [29]. While post-migration stressors seem to be of particular significance for longer-term mental health compared to premigration experiences [30, 31], premigration traumatic events do still exert influence, especially on post-traumatic rather than depressive symptoms [28, 29].

Case Study 2: Challenges of Care for Unaccompanied Young People

Fahmo is a 17-year-old orphan from Somalia, a practicing Muslim, who arrived in the UK as an unaccompanied asylum seeker. Fahmo arrived in the UK 3 years ago, at age 14, with her cousin, a Somali with British citizenship. Fahmo was abandoned shortly after arrival and placed in foster care with a white British family and enrolled in a secondary school in a small town with very few asylum seekers. The school had little support for new arrivals, so she was placed into mainstream classes despite speaking very little English and having little formal education. She felt "stupid" and was teased for wearing a headscarf; she felt unsafe at school and retaliated with verbally threatening behavior to classmates and carers.

Fahmo's foster placement broke down because of her behavior and she was moved to an emergency placement with another family in a large city. Her new foster mother, although not Muslim, took her to the mosque and Somali cultural center. Fahmo was placed in a new school where many students were migrants and had interventions in place to support these children to integrate at school. For example, Fahmo was "buddied" with a girl whose family had arrived 10 years earlier from Somalia, enabling her to join a wider friendship group. The school also had dedicated language support staff, who gradually integrated her into mainstream classes with the support of a teaching assistant. Fahmo's academic performance improved, although she still struggled with sleep, concentration, and motivation and often seemed distracted. Fahmo eventually accepted the offer of therapy sessions with the school counselor and began to develop a trusting relationship. She stopped wearing her headscarf and reduced attendance at the mosque and dressed similar to her new white and acculturated Somali friends.

One year later she was moved again to a Somali placement in a nearby town, as her foster family had only intended to offer an emergency placement. Fahmo needed to move school and end the counseling sessions due to distance. She found the new foster parents conservative and felt pressure to attend the mosque and dress more traditionally. Her behavior became increasingly challenging, and she was suspended from school for taking drugs. The pastoral support teacher had concerns that Fahmo might be experiencing symptoms of post-traumatic stress disorder. He tried to encourage Fahmo to accept a referral to child and adolescent mental health service, but she refused, saying there was no point, as she would only be moved somewhere else.

Chapter "School-Based Interventions" of this text by Miller, Bixby, and Ellis, offers an overview of tiered services operating in some schools. This case illustrates how different levels of intervention may be required at different stages of a young person's recovery. Case Example 2 illustrates how difficult repeated moves, although sometimes unavoidable, can have profound implications for mental health, particularly when young people are navigating the parallel challenges of moving on from a traumatic past, while simultaneously developing their identity and integrating into a new context. For young people already struggling to trust others, residential disruption can rapidly exhaust any remaining motivation to build new relationships with peers, care providers, and professionals or to engage in services that are offered. Such moves can also impact professionals' views and the services offered; they may become disheartened after being rendered unable to complete a course of therapy and may be reluctant to offer any interventions requiring a sustained commitment such as trauma-focused work, where environmental stability is important to safe and successful treatment.

Solutions

Principles of Mental Health Intervention

The majority of studies on risks for mental health problems have identified individual-level risk factors, with much less exploration of factors operating at family, community, and societal levels [2, 3]. These limitations in the evidence base are unfortunate, given the increasing recognition of the potential benefits of multimodal interventions, which could be better targeted with a more nuanced understanding of risks beyond the individual domain for each child. A multimodal intervention could, for example, address a range of problems influencing the young person negatively including psychological health, socioeconomic adversity, physical health, and community integration [32, 33]. Multimodal interventions targeting social and family adversity and structural inequalities, through community- or school-based intervention, offer promise, as discussed in Tyrer and Fazel [33] and Fazel et al. [34], a review of school-based interventions in low-income countries, many of which addressed the needs of refugee children.

However, such interventions may have different effects depending upon the context in which they are applied. For example, the classroom-based intervention (CBI) for children exposed to potentially traumatic events had differing results when evaluated in Burundi [35], Indonesia [36], Nepal [37], and Sri Lanka [38]; children in more settled contexts seemed to benefit more from the intervention [34]. Interventions may be universal, for example, delivered to a whole class; although such interventions are typically low cost to deliver, they also have many limitations to their effectiveness [33, 34, 39]. While they may have a role in the promotion of positive mental health, psychoeducation, and addressing minor difficulties, they are unlikely to be effective for children with serious psychological problems.

An alternative, more targeted, strategy is to deliver a group intervention to young people identified as being at increased risk. Such individuals could be identified either by the use of screening questionnaires, for example, for PTSD symptoms, or classification by the quantity or nature of adversities they have experienced, for example, children bereaved during conflict.

A key issue limiting recovery in displaced communities is that of stigma, relating to the distressing events themselves, especially in the case of sexual violence, and to the psychological sequelae of the events, as well as reluctance to seek help from mental health services. Effective interventions need to tackle the impact of shame at an individual and family level and stigmatization and discrimination operating at community and societal levels [40]. Without work to reduce stigma and optimize acceptability of interventions, available therapeutic resources will not be widely accessed by those in need.

Task shifting describes a human resource approach by which tasks are delegated to those with less training or narrower training [4, 41], which can enable the translation of interventions into settings where the existing skill mix or resource availability could not otherwise facilitate provision. Thus, lay workers with little or no training or experience in psychological treatment, but who show appropriate attributes and potential, receive training in specific skills to deliver treatment or prevention programs within their communities [42]. There is also an increasing interest in the utility of transdiagnostic or core element approaches in psychological intervention [43], whereby a modular approach is taken to delivering an evidence-based treatment to match a client's specific profile of needs. This approach is discussed in more detail in the chapter, "CBT with Immigrant Youth," by Thordarson, Keller, Sullivan, Trafalis, and Friedberg. These approaches may hold particular promise for scaling-up interventions in LMIC contexts, as they reduce

Table 2 Interventions with evidence for effectiveness in varying cultural contexts

	Target population	Mental health model	Countries delivered in	Outcomes
Jordans et al. [45]	Children in four conflict-affected countries	Multilayered psychosocial and mental healthcare delivery framework	Burundi, Sri Lanka, Indonesia, and Sudan	High levels of client satisfaction, moderate posttreatment problem reduction
Fox [46]	Southeast Asian refugees	School-based group CBT	USA	Reduced depressive symptoms
Robjant and Fazel [47]	Romania, Sudanese, Rwandan, Somalian, Sir Lankan	Narrative Exposure Therapy	Romania, Uganda, Rwanda, Germany, Norway, Sri Lanka	NET led to significant reductions in depression, physical health, and PTSD symptoms

the need for providers to be trained in different treatments and allow for more flexibility around ascribing a "correct" diagnosis before starting therapeutic work [44]. Table 2 gives examples of psychotherapeutic interventions found to be effective in refugee populations.

Models of Service Delivery in High-Income Settings

Practice and service delivery models are very different not only country by country but also region by region, such that it is rarely possible to give a unifying description of how a particular country approaches the treatment of refugee mental health. This differentiation necessarily reflects diverse needs and populations. For example, port regions often have a high concentration of asylum seekers, while economically deprived areas may be chosen by governments for "dispersal" of asylum seekers, because they have available and affordable housing. However, they may not have prior ethnic diversity, and staff may be inexperienced with cross-cultural work [48].

There is a range of different models of service delivery. In many areas, particularly where there are few asylum seekers, or organizational structures are inflexible, asylum seekers must access care through general mental health services. While they are less likely to see clinicians with expertise in working with interpreters, cross-cultural assessment, or post-traumatic stress, they may receive better care if their presentations are not of the classic triad affecting refugee populations, namely, PTSD, depression, and anxiety. Specialist mental health teams in refugee or transcultural care, offering direct access to appropriate psychological intervention, are more likely to be found in areas of higher refugee concentration. In other areas, services may be decentralized and delivered in a community-based or school-based format; the informality and flexibility of such services may improve their acceptability and accessibility for asylum seekers [33].

Case Study 3: Interagency Working to Meet Complex Family Needs

Noor fled Syria with her two children, Saeed, 4, and Sami, 14, after her husband was killed in front of the family. She is staying with her cousin, Bana, who was already resident in a high-income country, and is seeking asylum. Noor has developed PTSD. Saeed is showing developmentally regressive behaviors and encopresis, which Bana cannot tolerate. Sami is anxious and withdrawn. Bana helps Noor visit her general practitioner to discuss Saeed's encopresis. The general practitioner calls in the health visitor based at the practice to meet Noor while she is there. She offers a home visit to assess Saeed. There, she meets Sami and becomes concerned about his and Noor's mental health. She helps them make appointments at the practice and asks the general practitioner to arrange interpreters to allow Noor privacy to speak without Bana's presence. She suggests to the GP that Sami may be able to access counseling through a service offered in his school by visiting therapists from a voluntary organization. Sami agrees to try this, as he doesn't want to burden Bana with taking him to appointments. Noor is referred for specialist psychological therapy. Her general practitioner reviews her once a month, as there is a three-month waiting list for therapy; in the meantime, the health visitor builds a good relationship with Noor by fortnightly visits, and they make progress together in addressing Saeed's difficulties. Noor is pleased when she meets her own therapist, as she seems to understand that everyone in the family needs to get better together. She keeps her promise to call Sami's therapist and the health visitor before their next session, and Noor feels relieved when she offers to call a meeting for all the professionals involved with the family.

A particular challenge in providing quality care for refugees lies in meeting the needs of multiple generations with mental health needs, while not overburdening families with multiple appointments and professionals, and ensuring effective inter agency communication. While such interagency liaison can seem extremely time-consuming, ultimately once strong links are established between services, such relationships are reciprocally helpful. Most importantly, families have a much more positive experience of authorities and services, and there is recognition of how interrelated both distress and recovery are between family members.

Challenges and Opportunities in Low-Income Settings

The Mental Health Gap Action Program (mhGAP) is the World Health Organization's (WHO) program aiming to raise mental health in the political agenda and reduce the treatment gap between those in need and those in receipt of mental health interventions, with a particular focus on LMIC settings [49–51] where the dual challenges of economic disadvantage and instability affect care provision and there is a pressing need for scaling up of effective interventions [52]. Stability of residency is a particular problem in areas where ongoing unrest leads to multiple relocations, as affected populations are not resident for long enough for efficient, sustainable healthcare provision to be established. Although urgent physical and psychological care is patchily available in humanitarian contexts, typically through nongovernmental organization (NGO) provision, there is an increasing focus on local capacity building by using overseas expertise to train community workers, which is likely to be more sustainable, cost-effective, ethical, and acceptable to service users than models where non-local experts deliver short-term interventions [52]. This allows interventions to nest within the cultural and local context, offers employment to local people, and removes the constraints of delivering interventions through an interpreter.

A range of different models of care may be suitable in low-income settings, including group-based delivery, school-based interventions, and individual interventions [5]. Both individual and group therapy delivered by lay therapists will be illustrated in Case Examples 4 and 5 to highlight important considerations for successfully establishing sustainable services.

Narrative Exposure Therapy (NET) is an example of an individual intervention for post-traumatic symptoms, which has an increasingly strong evidence base for use in the LMIC context with forcibly displaced populations [47, 53, 54]. KidNET developed for children, and NET for adolescents and adults, have also been used with good results in HIC [47]. The features of NET which make it particularly well suited to LMIC are its relative brevity, suitability for multiple traumatic events, acceptability to cultures with an oral rather than written tradition, and suitability for those with low literacy. Moreover, it can be taught relatively quickly to local staff without broad prior mental health training.

Case Study 4: Individual Intervention in a Low-Income Setting

Joy is a 33-year-old teacher, living in a refugee camp in Uganda. While many of the displaced people residing in the camp are Ugandan, conflict in South Sudan has brought successive waves of refugees to live alongside existing camp residents. Joy has been trained by an overseas NGO to use NET and she works primarily with children. She uses her classroom out of hours as a quiet, private location that it is easy for children to access.

One of Joy's clients is Amina, a teenage refugee from South Sudan who experienced multiple traumatic events. Using flowers and stones she collects from the surrounding area, Joy works with Amina to create a lifeline of the important events in her life. Each traumatic event, represented as stones, is retold in great detail, as Joy helps Amina to contextualize and order her memories. During this work Joy aims to reduce Amina's fear of the memory by helping Amina integrate fragmented memories into the broader context in which the events occurred. Joy sees children individually and never works with more than a few individuals at a time. Owing to unexpected relocation of refugees at any time and low resources, sessions are held weekly and can take place twice a week, often not needing more than 8–10 sessions per child. Joy's clients do not pay for treatment, but Joy receives a small monthly stipend, which comes from matched funding paid by the NGO to supplement the contribution made by her country's government to the therapists' salaries. She also tries to meet with the other local women who were trained to deliver NET for peer supervision.

Enthusiastic and respected lay workers such as Joy, firmly nested within their own community, are a vital component of sustainable interventions. The time and expertise needed for supervision must be factored into programs being established in low-income settings, especially as local staff may have limited therapeutic experience, current and past adversities of their own, and a high workload. Ensuring that local therapists feel motivated and supported and have opportunities for professional development is an important factor in staff retention and preventing burnout.

Case Study 5: Group Intervention and Local Capacity Building

Tariq is a teacher working in Gaza at a secondary school with many forcibly displaced children attending. The school took part in NGO training to run psychosocial school group interventions with children showing symptoms of PTSD and associated psychopathology. The intervention could be administered by local lay therapists without formal mental health training. Teachers are asked to identify children who display behaviors such as jumpy and startled responses, flashbacks, low self-esteem, high absenteeism, and conflict with peers and teachers. The intervention is manual based and consists of 10 sessions incorporating cognitive behavioral techniques over a 10-week period. The main aim of the intervention is to educate children on the common symptoms associated with exposure to potentially traumatic events and strategies that might help them gain more control over these symptoms. Strategies such as drama, movement, music, art, and play therapy are used to promote the children's natural resilience in an effort to foster a more positive outlook over the course of the program. The program also endeavors to involve parents and the local community through engagement, education, and outreach so that the students are surrounded by a strong support structure and people who understand and trust the program.

Staff from the NGO keep in regular touch with Tariq by video calls and visit the school quarterly for the first year to support therapists to assess their outcomes and offer opportunities for supervision and skill development.

Well-targeted group intervention can be a positive solution in a resource-poor context, and teachers are ideally placed to identify struggling young people most in need of this step-up from a universal intervention to a more selected one. While clinicians are appropriately keen to achieve as full a recovery as possible for each individual patient, in terms of public mental health, a reduction in symptoms rather than a full remission is still a worthwhile (albeit suboptimal) outcome, which may produce sufficient change to allow reasonable engagement in education, employment, family, and community life. Ongoing investment by the training body into supporting and further skill building allows the intervention to embed successfully in the local context until therapists become confident enough to offer each other peer supervision on a longer-term basis. Evaluation of outcomes is very important, to ensure that any adaptations for the local context have not adversely impacted effectiveness and that therapists are able to maintain fidelity and competence in the intervention as external support is tapered off.

Conclusion and Future Directions

Delivering effective psychological treatment is fraught with challenges in any context of forced displacement. Rapid and equitable access to evidence-based, culturally sensitive mental health interventions is an aspiration which has yet to come to fruition in the vast majority of settings and services. Standalone psychological intervention would benefit from parallel attention to reducing broader stressors and mobilizing positive resources and sources of support. Clinicians working therapeutically with forcibly displaced populations risk being overwhelmed and ineffective unless they forge supportive reciprocal relationships with other services meeting refugees' social, educational, and legal needs.

The priorities in service development in both high- and low-income contexts are in the implementation of evidence-based interventions, while evaluating the impact upon effectiveness of any changes that are made in order to adapt such interventions to the local context [55]. In both settings, the participation of service users in research and service redesign is vital not only to optimize acceptability but also to embed services within the communities they serve. Clinicians can be strong advocates for change to policies which are anecdotally harmful, most particularly for vulnerable populations with little opportunity for self-advocacy, such as refugees. The effective targeting of healthcare resources for the most needy individuals and families is key in both contexts, which requires the development of appropriate triaging systems and networks with other agencies, both as sources of referral and for signposting those not requiring specialist support. While much progress has been made in local capacity building in low-income settings, the mental health treatment gap between those in need and those in receipt of healthcare is enormous, and reducing disparities in treatment availability for mental versus physical healthcare is a key sustainable development priority [56].

References

1. Betancourt TS, Khan KT. The mental health of children affected by armed conflict: protective processes and pathways to resilience. Int Rev Psychiatry. 2008;20(3):317–28.
2. Fazel M, Reed RV, Panter-Brick C, Stein A. Mental health of displaced and refugee children resettled in high-income countries: risk and protective factors. Lancet. 2012;379(9812): 266–82.
3. Reed RV, Fazel M, Jones L, Panter-Brick C, Stein A. Mental health of displaced ad refugee children resettled in low-income and middle-income countries: risk and protective factors. Lancet. 2012;379(9812):250–65.
4. Kakuma R, Minas H, Van-Ginneken N, Dal-Poz MR, Desiraju K, Morris JE, et al. Human resources for mental health care: current situation and strategies for action. Lancet. 2011;378(9803):1654–63.
5. Kieling C, Baker-Henningham H, Belfer M, Conti G, Ertem I, Omigbodun O, et al. Child and adolescent mental health worldwide: evidence for action. Lancet. 2011;378(9801):1515–25.
6. Zimmerman C, Kiss L, Hossain M. Migration and health: a framework for 21st century policy-making. PLoS Med. 2011;8(5), e1001034.
7. UNHCR. UNHCR global trends: forced displacement in 2014. Geneva: UNHCR; 2015.
8. Hodes M, Jagdev D, Chandra N, Cunniff A. Risk and resilience for psychological distress amongst unaccompanied asylum seeking adolescents. J Child Psychol Psychiatry. 2008;49(7): 723–32.
9. Ferguson A. Refugee camp for Syrians in Jordan evolves as a do-it-yourself city. The New York Times; 2014.
10. Jacobsen LB. Finding means: UNRWA's financial Situation and the living conditions of Palestinian refugees. Summary Report. Oslo, FAFO; 2000.
11. Crisp J. A state of insecurity: the political economy of violence in Kenya's refugee camps. Afr Aff. 2000;99:601–32.
12. Miller KE, Rasmussen A. War exposure, daily stressors, and mental health in conflict ad post-conflict settings: bridging the divide between trauma-focused and psychosocial frameworks. Soc Sci Med. 2010;70(1):7–16.
13. Rousseau C, Heusch N. The trip: a creative expression project for refugee and immigrant children. J Am Art Ther Assoc. 2000;17:31–40.
14. Fazel M, Karunakara UK, Newnham EA. Detention, denial, and death: migrant hazards for refugee children. Lancet Glob Health. 2014;2(6):313–4.
15. Suárez-Orozco C, Todorova ILG, Louie J. Making up for lost time: the experience of separation and reunification among immigrant families. Fam Process. 2002;41(4):625–43.
16. Menjívar C. Transnational parenting and immigration law: Central Americans in the United States. J Ethn Migr Stud. 2012;38(2):301–22.
17. Molina KE, Kohm LM. "Are we there yet?" Immigration reform for children left behind. Berkeley La Raza Law J. 2013;23:77–108.
18. Joffe-Block J. New immigration policy aims to limit family separation; 2013. Retrieved from http://www.fronterasdesk.org/content/new-immigration-policy-aims-limit-family-separation
19. Ambert AM, Krull C. Changing families: relationships in context. Upper Saddle River, NJ: Pearson; 2006.
20. Bernhard JK, Landolt P, Goldring L. Transnational, multi-local motherhood: experiences of separation and reunification among Latin American families in Canada. 36 pp. CERIS Working Paper Number 40, July 2005. Published by Joint Centre of Excellence for Research on Immigration and Settlement, Toronto (CERIS), Toronto, ON, Canada; 2005.
21. Dreby J. Children and power in Mexican transnational families. J Marriage Fam. 2007;69: 1050–64.
22. Wong BP. Immigration, globalization and the Chinese American family. In: Lansford JE, Deater-Deckard KD, Bornstein MH, editors. Immigrant families in contemporary society. New York: Guilford; 2006. p. 212–29.

23. Streamlining legal immigration; 2015. Retrieved from http://www.whitehouse.gov/issues/immigration/streamlining-immigration
24. United Nations Development Programme. Human development report 2009—overcoming barriers: human mobility and development. New York: Author; 2009.
25. Suárez-Orozco C, Bang HJ, Kim HY. I felt like my heart was staying behind: psychological implications of family separations and reunifications for immigrant youth. J Adolesc Res. 2011;26(2):222–57.
26. Fazel M, Wheeler J, Danesh J. Prevalence of serious mental disorders in 7000 refugees resettled in western countries: a systematic review. Lancet. 2005;365(9467):1309–14.
27. Hjern A, Angel B. Organized violence and mental health of refugee children in exile: a six-year follow-up. Acta Paediatr. 2000;89(6):722–7.
28. Sack WH, Clarke G, Him C, Dickason D, Goff B, Lanham K, Kinzie JD. A 6-year follow-up study of Cambodian refugee adolescents traumatized as children. J Am Acad Child Adolesc Psychiatry. 1993;32(2):431–7.
29. Sack WH, Him C, Dickason D. Twelve-year follow-up study of Khmer youths who suffered massive war trauma as children. J Am Acad Child Adolesc Psychiatry. 1999;38(9):1173–9.
30. Montgomery E. Long-term effects of organized violence on young Middle Eastern refugees' mental health. Soc Sci Med. 2008;67(10):1596–603.
31. Montgomery E. Trauma and resilience in young refugees: a 9-year follow-up study. Dev Psychopathol. 2010;22(02):477–89.
32. Nickerson A, Bryant RA, Silove D, Steel Z. A critical review of psychological treatments of posttraumatic stress disorder in refugees. Clin Psychol Rev. 2011;31(3):399–417.
33. Tyrer R, Fazel M. School and community based interventions for refugee and asylum seeking children: a systematic review. PLoS One. 2014;9(2):e89359. doi:10.1371/journal.pone.0089359.
34. Fazel M, Patel V, Thomas S, Tol W. Mental health interventions in schools in low-income and middle-income countries. Lancet Psychiatry. 2014;1(5):388–98.
35. Jordans MJ, Tol WA, Susanty D, Ntamatumba P, Luitel NP, Komproe IH, de Jong JT. Implementation of a mental health care package for children in areas of armed conflict: a case study from Burundi, Indonesia, Nepal, Sri Lanka, and Sudan. PLoS Med. 2013;10(1): e1001371. doi:10.1371/journal.pmed.1001371.
36. Tol W, Komproe IH, Jordans MJD, Ndaisaba A, Ntamutumba P, Sipsma H, et al. School-based mental health interventions for children affected by political violence in Indonesia: a cluster randomised trial. J Am Med Assoc. 2008;300(6):655–62.
37. Jordans MJ, Komproe IH, Tol WA, Kohrt BA, Luitel NP, Macy RD, De-Jong JT. Evaluation of a classroom-based psychosocial intervention in conflict-affected Nepal: a cluster randomized controlled trial. J Child Psychol Psychiatry. 2010;51(7):818–26.
38. Tol WA, Komproe IH, Jordans MJD, Vallipuram A, Sipsma H, Sivayokan S, et al. Outcomes and moderators of a preventative school-based mental health interventions for children affected by war in Sri Lanka: a cluster randomized trial. World Psychiatry. 2012;11(2):114–22.
39. Betancourt TS, Meyers-Ohki SE, Charrow AP, Tol WA. Interventions for children affected by war: an ecological perspective on psychosocial support and mental health care. Harv Rev Psychiatry. 2013;21(2):70–91.
40. Saraceno B, Van Ommeren M, Batniji R, Cohen A, Gureje O, Mahoneye J, et al. Barriers to improvement of mental health services in low-income and middle-income countries. Lancet. 2007;370(9593):1164–74.
41. Fulton BD, Scheffler RM, Sparkes SP, Auh EY, Vujicic M, Soucat A. Health workforce skill mix and task shifting in low income countries: a review of recent evidence. Hum Resour Health. 2011;9:1. doi:10.1186/1478-4491-9-1.
42. Murray LK, Dorsey S, Haroz E, Lee C, Alsiary MM, Haydary A, et al. A common elements treatment approach for adult mental health problems in low- and middle-income countries. Cogn Behav Pract. 2014;21(2):111–23.
43. Chorpita BF, Daleiden EL, Weisz JR. Identifying and selecting the common elements of evidence based interventions: a distillation and matching model. Ment Health Serv Res. 2005;7(1):5–20.

44. Bolton PF, Lee C, Haroz EE, Murra L, Dorsey S, Robison C, et al. A transdiagnostic community-based mental health treatments for comorbid disorders: development and outcome of a randomized controlled trial among Burmese Refugees in Thailand. PLoS Med. 2014;11(11):e1001757. doi:10.1371/journal.pmed.1001757.
45. Jordans MJD, Komproe IH, Tol WA, Susanty D, Vallipuram A, Ntamatumba P, et al. Practice-driven evaluation of a multi-layered psychosocial care package for children in areas of armed conflict. Community Ment Health J. 2011;47:267–77.
46. Fox, P. G., Rossetti, J., Burns, K. R., & Popovich, J. (2005). Southeast Asian refugee children: a school-based mental health intervention. The international journal of psychiatric nursing research, 11(1), 1227–1236.
47. Robjant K, Fazel M. The emerging evidence for Narrative Exposure Therapy: a review. Clin Psychol Rev. 2010;30(8):1030–9.
48. Ehntholt KA, Yule W. Practitioner review: assessment and treatment of refugee children and adolescents who have experienced war-related trauma. J Child Psychol Psychiatry. 2006;47(12):1197–210.
49. Patel V, Araya R, Chatterjee S, Chisholm D, Cohen A, De Silva M, et al. Treatment and prevention of mental disorders in low-income and middle-income countries. Lancet. 2007; 370(9591):991–1005.
50. Patel V, Collins PY, Copeland J, Kakuma R, Katontoka S, Lamichhane J, et al. The movement for global mental health. Br J Psychiatry. 2011;198(2):88–90.
51. WHO. Mental Health Gap Action Programme (mhGap): scaling up care for mental, neurological and substance use disorders. Geneva: World Health Organisation; 2008.
52. Eaton J, McCay L, Semrau M, Chatterjee S, Baingana F, Araya R, Ntulo C, et al. Scale up of services for mental health in low-income and middle-income countries. Lancet. 2011; 378(9802):1592–603.
53. Catani C, Kohiladevy MR, Schauer M, Elbert ET, Neuner F. Treating children traumatized by war and Tsunami: a comparison between exposure therapy and meditation-relaxation in North-East Sri Lanka. BMC Psychiatry. 2009;9:22. doi:10.1186/1471-244X-9-22.
54. Ertl V, Pfeiffer A, Schauer E, Elbert T, Neuner F. Community-implemented trauma therapy for former child soldiers in Northern Uganda: a randomized controlled trial. J Am Med Assoc. 2011;306(5):503–12.
55. Tol WA, Barbui C, Galappatti A, Silove D, Betancourt TS, Souza R, et al. Mental health and psychosocial support in humanitarian settings: linking practice and research. Lancet. 2011;378(9802):1581–91.
56. Thornicroft G, Patel V. Including mental health among the new sustainable development goals. BMJ. 2014;349(7972):5.

Immigrant Youth and Navigating Unique Systems That Interact with Treatment

David E. Reed II, Marilee Ruebsamen, James Livingston, and Fazia Eltareb

Abstract

Understanding the challenges that immigrant children and their families face as part of the immigration process to the United States of America (USA) is a reflection of their circumstances of arrival and is essential for providing clinical services. Immigrant youth and their families may arrive as refugees, political asylum seekers, or both. Children and youth are particularly vulnerable to being part of a child-trafficking forced migration. Because of these unique circumstances, case management and service coordination often become a significant part of treatment. In many cases, simultaneous coordination between traditional patient care (i.e., general practitioner, psychiatrist, and psychologist), a case manager, a resettlement agency, an attorney, and specific governmental agencies is indicated. Adding to these complications are possible language and cultural barriers that come with migration. With these barriers, children may become cultural brokers to their parents, which has its advantages and disadvantages. Explanations of these systems and specific barriers that immigrant youth and mental health workers may encounter are presented. Case studies are presented in order to help illustrate how clinicians can help patients overcome these barriers and have a successful immigration experience.

D.E. Reed II, M.S. (✉) • F. Eltareb, M.S.
Palo Alto University, 1791 Arastradero Road, Palo Alto, CA 94304, USA
e-mail: dreed@paloaltou.edu; feltareb@paloaltou.edu

M. Ruebsamen, Ph.D.
Abbey Psychological Services, 940 Saratoga Ave., Ste. 200, San Jose, CA 95129, USA
e-mail: drmarilee@abbeypsychservices.com

J. Livingston, Ph.D.
Center for Survivors of Torture, Asian Americans for Community Involvement,
2400 Moorpark Ave., San Jose, CA 95129, USA
e-mail: james.livingston@aaci.org

© Springer International Publishing Switzerland 2016
S.G. Patel, D. Reicherter (eds.), *Psychotherapy for Immigrant Youth*,
DOI 10.1007/978-3-319-24693-2_9

Keywords
Refugees • Political asylum seekers • Child trafficking • Cultural brokers
• Resettlement agency

Immigrant Youth and Navigating Unique Social Systems That Interact with Treatment

Understanding the challenges that immigrant children and their families face as part of the immigration process to the USA is a reflection of their circumstances of arrival and is essential for providing clinical services. For some immigrants, the dangers are minimal; for others, legal status in immigration is a matter of life and death. All immigrants by definition have left their home and most of what composes it: family members, friends, places, people, customs, culture, and often language. A great majority of people immigrating to the USA do so voluntarily. Those who do so are motivated by the ambition of a better life than the one they would have had if they had remained in their home country [1]. It is the adults, however, who make such decisions, and children must follow, not always willingly. It can be a wrenching experience for adolescents to lose their peer group and be thrown into entirely new circumstances [2]. Fortunately, research suggests that resilience in children is more of a rule rather than an exception [3], enabling them to recover from the losses, learn the new language when necessary, and adjust to the culture in which they now live much more rapidly than their parents or other adult caretakers. Not all adults immigrate by choice, however: some immigrate by force. The migration of human beings due to threat has a long history, wherein the potential advantages of a better life outweigh the dangers of the move [4].

There are three broad categories under which individuals arrive, either by choice or by force: refugee, trafficked, and voluntary immigration. A fourth category, asylum seekers, represents those who are attempting to gain the designation as a refugee [2, 5]. As a result, the US government has specific mechanisms in place that work with individuals who fit into any of the above immigration categories. Not only do they involve the ability for individuals to receive health care, it also includes a monetary stipend and avenues to obtain legal representation and housing.

The circumstances of arrival are qualitatively different. Depending on these circumstances, different trauma histories of patients may be considered, as well as which systems mental health workers may encounter. As such, delineating the four different pathways of arrival and the unique systems that correspond to these pathways is crucial to understanding how they interact with treatment. After describing the process and circumstances of arrival, we will discuss likely systems mental health workers will encounter, barriers to treatment, and how immigrant youth may become cultural brokers between their new environment and the older generation. Case studies are presented in order to help illustrate how clinicians can help patients overcome these barriers and have a successful immigration experience.

Refugees

In 1950, the United Nations (UN) defined a refugee as someone who fled their home country after being persecuted for their beliefs and who is also unable to seek refuge with their country's government [6]. The term refugee also serves as a legal definition of status within the US legal system [7]. Those seeking refuge and who do not directly immigrate to the USA most often travel to a safer country than their own where they apply for refugee status with the UN or at a US embassy. When the search for safety leads an immigrant family to a developing country, they may find themselves in an informal refugee camp lacking basic assistance such as electricity and water (see Fazel et al. [8]). Indeed, low-income countries see the highest level of immigration [8].

Refugees in the USA outnumber any other country in the world [9]. In fiscal year 2013 alone, 24,718 children (35 % of total) entered the USA as a refugee [10]. They depart their home country due to the psychological and/or physical harm they endured, often due to religious or political views [4]. War, crimes against humanity, political strife, religious beliefs, gender, and ethnicity may all play a role in their forced migration [2]. These individuals are escaping a way of life that may include fear, intimidation, marginalization, and a limited future. Their level of fear and anxiety and desire for a better life outweigh their feelings of comfort in family, friends, and culture in their home country.

It is important to understand that refugee youth are in their current state of crisis at least partially due to their worldviews (i.e., culturally determined beliefs that encompass assumptions about reality [11]). They are in many cases persecuted for these beliefs (e.g., sexual orientation and gender), resulting in their forced migration. Janoff-Bulman's [12, 13] shattered assumptions theory and, more recently, Abdollahi et al.'s [14] anxiety buffer disruption theory (ABDT) have provided compelling evidence that trauma symptoms are a direct result from these worldviews no longer having the ability to protect an individual from the world's dangerous realities. ABDT, formed out of terror management theory (TMT) [15], is particularly compelling as it has provided direct experimental evidence that worldview disruption leads to traumatic symptoms [11, 14], and those with high traumatic symptoms lack an anxiety buffer or are unable to utilize it [16–18]. According to TMT, worldviews play an integral part in protecting human beings from the terror that comes from the realization that we all will one day perish. Furthermore, by living up to these worldviews, human beings gain a sense of self-esteem (for review, see Pyszczynski et al. [19]). This places refugee youth at particular risk as their worldviews may have been consistently derogated. Their sense of safety and belief that the world is a safe place (cf. [13]) may be shattered. They may not trust others, which can serve as a barrier to mental health treatment [2]. Overcoming these issues of trust may provide a mediator between patient engagement and improved mental health. Piecing these worldviews back together may be an integral part of helping youth gain a sense of purpose and meaning in the world, thus improving self-esteem.

Case Study

"Henri" was a 17-year-old boy, originally from Burundi, who arrived as a
refugee in the USA from Tunisia almost 2 months prior to his clinical intake.
He was brought to that appointment by his social worker from his resettlement agency, Catholic Charities, one of the largest nonprofit organizations in
the USA with many programs, among which is the resettlement of refugee,
unaccompanied minors. Because he was a minor without relatives in the USA,
that agency was functioning as his guardian. "Henri" was born and reared in
Burundi with his 11 siblings. He realized and communicated to his parents
that he was gay at an early age, whereupon he began experiencing rejection by
his family. Growing up, he was mocked, insulted, and beaten, both at home
and in the community. About 18 months prior to his intake, his parents found
him kissing another boy, and they called the police. Because homosexual acts
are a crime in Burundi punishable by up to 2 years imprisonment, Henri
escaped and traveled to Tunisia, where his boyfriend had already relocated.
There, guided by his boyfriend, he went to the US embassy and filled out the
paperwork to apply for refugee status in the USA. He lived in Tunisia for over
a year when his boyfriend was accepted as a refugee and left for the
USA. Feeling abandoned and alone, "Henri" attempted suicide by drinking
poison. He was briefly hospitalized, and a few months thereafter he was
granted refugee status and traveled to the USA.

Asylum Seekers

Asylum seekers are defined as individuals who have yet to attain refugee status but
are actively seeking out this designation [2, 5]. Asylum is offered when the applicant has been persecuted or is in danger of persecution due to race, nationality,
religion, political opinion, or membership in a social group [20]. The UN has a
formalized international policy for individuals seeking the official refugee designation [5], but this is relegated to participating countries. Within this process, the
legitimacy of the danger they would face should they return home is investigated,
and if found to be valid, they are recognized as being refugees and await placement
in a receiving country (see UNHCR [21] for detailed information on this process).

Within the USA, any individual who is seeking this designation must be referred to
the US Refugee Admissions Program (USRAP) which handles the application process for each individual [20]. Even if immigrants arrive in the USA in a manner other
than to seek asylum (e.g., student, tourist, work visas, or surreptitiously), they are still
able to apply. The US government, through the USRAP, treats those individuals using
the same process as those who came to the USA seeking a refugee designation, which
includes an interview with an asylum officer where an applicant is required to produce
evidence of their identity, group membership, and persecution in their home country.

While other countries have different application processes, the USA uses Form
I-589, Application for Asylum and for Withholding of Removal [20], which asks

applicants to detail the circumstances of their persecution [22]. This form is a lengthy, 15-page form that asks for detailed information about the applicant and his or her spouse, children, and parents. Included in this background information are previous addresses and employment. Depending on the circumstances, the most stressful part of the application process may be the fact that it asks for detailed explanations as to why the applicant is seeking asylum. In other words, the form asks for a trauma history. In a clinical setting, mental health workers are taught to build rapport and create a zone of trust before delving into such histories. Here, the US government is concerned about no such thing. Not only can the recall of events be stressful, but the fact that other legal-status opportunities are dependent on this process can also be anxiety provoking. For instance, in order for an individual to be able to bring his or her family to the USA or to become a permanent resident, asylum must be granted [20]. This process would not necessarily apply to children, but it would affect their parents and any adult children. In turn, this may affect children's emotional well-being, making this process important for both parents and children [23].

If their application was with the US State Department, they await their security background check and for a placement opening somewhere in the USA. Unfortunately, they have no choice as to where they will initially live. This uncertainty can be an anxiety-provoking time for the children who are awaiting their own status or the status of their parents. Complicating the situation is that whether the application takes place through the USA or UN, both processes are lengthy and often lasts for years. Once granted refugee status and after 5 years as a permanent resident, a refugee family has the ability to apply for citizenship through the naturalization process [24].

Case Study

"Humberto" is a 45-year-old father of three who arrived in the USA from Nicaragua almost 5 years before the initial clinical intake, having been granted asylum 6 months before the appointment. He entered the USA as a tourist and applied for asylum upon his arrival, but his asylum approval was delayed, initially due to difficulty in documenting his persecution. Accordingly, the asylum officer referred his application to a hearing, and because of the magnitude of the backlog of applicants, his hearing was not held for another 3 years. He had been managing a company in Nicaragua for 6 years when a drug cartel demanded payment in exchange for allowing the company to continue doing business. Initially, Humberto made the payments, but he soon ran out of money. When his family was threatened, he resigned his position. However, threats continued, so he moved his family to another city. Five months after their move, they were discovered and the threats resumed. His adult sons moved out of the country, and Humberto left for the USA. During the 3 years of waiting for his hearing, he talked with his wife and daughter, who was a minor, daily. His wife and daughter continued to move every few months to avoid discovery by cartel members, creating a constant sense of threat and anxiety in both his wife and daughter. They had arrived from Nicaragua less than a month prior to the intake and were now in the process of reconnecting as a family.

If asylum is granted, the asylee has the same legal status and governmental support as an arriving refugee. That is, they will be eligible to apply for work authorization, travel abroad, bring their family members to the USA [7], and receive the monthly refugee stipend. If there is insufficient evidence or there is some other technical/legal issue that makes the case unclear, the asylum officer will refer the applicant to an immigration judge. Fewer than 30 % of recent applicants have been granted asylum [25]. If denied, many applicants have the opportunity to either file for an appeal or for a motion to reopen the case [26]. Which route an applicant should take will be explained by the denial letter the applicant receives [26]. While the USCIS tries to resolve appeals within 6 months, this is not guaranteed [26], possibly adding and prolonging the anxiety and stress that comes with this process. While waiting for the Immigration and Customs Enforcement process to slowly progress, the applicant can apply for work authorization after 150 days [20] but is not eligible for any public assistance [27]. It normally falls to religious charities and community not-for-profit organizations to support asylum seekers to the degree that they are able to do so. It is not uncommon for an asylum seeker to have no dependable source of food, shelter, clothing, and other basic necessities. This can result in added pressure and stress regarding the asylum process. Legal representation is not a right for an applicant, who must pay for the assistance of an immigration attorney, find one on a pro bono basis, or proceed without representation. These processes may be difficult for some to undertake. Mental health workers may find themselves helping their client process the thoughts and emotions that come with these applications along with helping them understand the forms. Youth may have a difficult time understanding why their parents are stressed, not recognizing the importance of this process. This is yet another way that working with refugee youth comes with a unique set of circumstances.

Youth may apply for asylum without an adult [28]. In fact, minors have the right to apply for asylum even if their parent is also applying for asylum, allowing for separate immigration processes [28]. The US government has guidelines in place for interviewers that are meant to take into account the child's developmental level [28]. While this may result in increased sensitivity to the child's mental health, these are not professional mental health care workers. Those working with youth in the mental health field may find themselves discussing with the child this interview process and how that negatively affected, or even re-traumatized, the child. Whether an adult or child, providing basic resources such as food and shelter may be the responsibility of an agency that specializes in such matters.

Resettlement Agency

When refugees are scheduled to travel to the USA, a nongovernmental resettlement agency becomes responsible for their preparation for arrival [29]. As the similarities between their home country and USA decrease, the difficulty of adjustment increases [30]. For refugees coming from developing countries, their transition to the USA can be tantamount to traveling centuries into the future, where their experiences include new modes of travel, technology, and attitudes about social issues. They may have no experience or exposure to the use of electrical appliances, indoor plumbing, and the like. Everything seems to be new and often bewildering. It is the task of the resettlement agencies to ease this transition [31].

While well intentioned, most resettlement agencies are underfunded and overwhelmed by the volume of refugees they serve. This commonly results in their providing the most minimal of services, sometimes even leaving it to newly arrived refugees to find their own housing within a month of their arrival. While the US government provides a financial stipend to refugees for 8 months following their arrival, the tasks that must be accomplished in that timeframe to become self-sufficient, such as learning English and developing skills for gainful employment, can be overwhelming. Such tasks may be daunting to someone who arrives well-functioning, eager, and culturally oriented. These tasks become even more difficult for those refugees who are traumatized by their experiences of persecution, flight from their home country, and their wait for placement while in a transitional country [32].

Child Trafficking

Another way children come to the USA is through the crime of human trafficking. The US government defines trafficking as the exploitation of others through "force, fraud, or coercion" for the purposes of sex or labor and describe it as a "modern form of slavery" [33]. Obtaining accurate numerical estimations on human trafficking is difficult; however, the US government reported that between 2003 and 2004 alone, 14,500 to 17,500 individuals were victims of human trafficking into the USA [34]. These individuals are not only going through the horror of forced sexual or labor activities, but this is occurring in an unfamiliar setting. The US government offers relief for such victims in the form of the T visa [35]. This application may be used by victims if they are willing to comply with law enforcement investigators regarding human trafficking perpetrators, although this is not required if the person is under the age of 18 or if they qualify as having symptoms of traumatic stress [35]. For mental health workers, this latter exemption may seem redundant with being a victim of human trafficking. Nevertheless, an outlet exists that can begin the process of providing a safe haven for these victims.

Part of the difficulty for clinicians working with this population is the coordination with multiple systems, particularly the legal system. Remaining within ethical boundaries, clinicians should be prepared to navigate the legal process with a client who may not understand the process in its entirety. Furthermore, new means of employment and new housing may be a top priority for these individuals in order to fully escape their previous life [32]. They also may be suffering from sexually transmitted infections [36]; therefore, coordinating with a primary care physician may be integral to providing excellent treatment. While navigating all of these systems is discussed further with more details, it should be evident that refugees, including trafficked children, are a unique population that requires qualitatively different treatment than traditional mental health treatment (e.g., weekly emotional processing for 1 h [37, 38]).

Case Study

"Anjali" was an 18-year-old single woman who arrived in the USA from India on a work visa. She was brought to the USA 2 years prior to the initial clinical intake by her employers, an Indian couple, to serve as a nanny. She was tearful and expressed desperation. Her employers paid her at a rate below minimum wage, allowed her no time off, and required her to pay them rent for her room. She was to be available 24 h per day for childcare, cooking, and cleaning. She was also treated with disrespect, often berated by her employers. They had accused her of stealing from them and had spread this rumor within their ethnic community so that she had no opportunity to find different employment. Despite their accusations, they continued to have her as a servant in their home.

Unaccompanied Minors

The final group discussed here are unaccompanied minors. These are children who have crossed into the USA without an adult or who have been abandoned by an adult [39]. Trafficked and unaccompanied children have no guardian in the USA and, if identified, must have a legal guardian assigned to them. Sometimes upon their arrival in the USA, they find that the parent with whom they sought to reunite is not interested in resuming their parenting. A variety of nonprofit organizations have undertaken that role, seeking to place as many as possible into foster homes [40]. Many, however, cannot be placed with foster parents and instead are placed into group homes designed for children without parents. When a nonprofit is unable to immediately identify housing, the child is placed into an Immigration and Customs Enforcement detention center until more suitable care can be identified [40]. As of 2014, under the Deferred Action for Childhood Arrivals (DACA), children who cross the border unaccompanied and who are registered as such have been granted a 2-year stay of deportation while their legal options can be explored [41]. If deemed qualified for asylum, they are allowed to remain in the USA until a decision is reached regarding their application. As of this writing, it is unclear how children who do not qualify for asylum will be handled if no relative can be identified in their home country.

In the USA, many of these children and their parents, typically from Mexico, Central America, and Caribbean countries, move fluidly across borders such that the term "transnational" has been used to describe their identification of their nationality [42]. Participation in their faith centers is often the unifying element between the cultures and their sense of identification [42].

Case Study

"Carlos" was a 16-year-old boy who arrived from his native Mexico 6 months prior to the initial clinical intake. He was brought into the clinic by his pro bono lawyer for a psychological evaluation for use in his application for asylum. He explained that his mother had left for the USA 2 years prior to his crossing the border, with the intent of securing employment and then sending for him. While waiting and living with his grandmother, he had repeatedly been approached by gang members seeking to recruit him. After several refusals, they began harassing him, threatening him and his grandmother, and twice beating him. He took refuge in a church and was not able to leave for nearly 1 year. Despite many harrowing experiences, he found his aunt, and through her, his mother. His mother unfortunately had made it clear that she was "very busy" and therefore he could not live with her. He was deferential and a bit shy. He explained through the interpreter that he wanted to attend school in the USA.

Upon the second meeting 5 weeks later, "Carlos'" presentation had markedly changed. He appeared to be depressed, was unkempt, and dressed in the manner typical of local gang members. He was either unresponsive to questions or surly when he did respond. He eventually explained that he had seen two members of the gang that had harassed him in Mexico while in a shopping center. He had managed to leave before they saw him but now was unable to leave his aunt's home, feeling just as imprisoned as he had in Mexico. Despite saying she would attend two pre-court family interviews, his mother appeared for neither. She also had failed to respond to his lawyer's messages encouraging her to appear at his upcoming asylum hearing. His mother did not attend the hearing, and his asylum application was denied. He disappeared and could not be found.

Simultaneous Navigation of Services

Often, immigrant youth face a new way of life while also dealing with past hardships, language barriers, and other acculturative stressors. An example of an agency seeking to serve refugees and asylum seekers is the Center for Survivors of Torture (CST) at Asian Americans for Community Involvement (AACI) in San Jose, CA. It is common for new clients to be exclusively focused on their basic needs such as food, housing, and employment and rightfully so. At the same time, these clients may not see a need for traditional mental health treatment. Many immigrants are wary of seeking help due to the stigmatization and fear of discrimination [43]. They also fear what may come of a mental health diagnosis [43]. While they may also fear the loss or separation of their children [43], the youth involved in these decisions may benefit greatly from services that focus on making connections within their respective communities (e.g., religious organizations) or broader-based communities (e.g., YMCA).

When staff recognizes that mental health treatment is needed, they often seek to overcome these barriers to treatment by focusing on aspects of case management. This often proves to be an impactful entry point for mental health treatment for many new clients. Case managers serve as social workers and play an integral role at CST, as they are often the persons who help new refugees orient themselves to life in the USA. Many immigrants are not aware of the many services that are in place designed to help individuals such as them. For example, many refugees qualify for reduced-cost bus passes, bagged lunches, and free groceries. Case managers can also help new arrivals get acquainted with the different immigration laws and suggest accessible attorneys who are experienced within the immigration process.

CST helps navigate multiple kinds of resources within the immigrant community even beyond immigration law. They are able to coordinate services with other organizations, such as Catholic Charities and the International Refugee Committee (IRC), both of which assist immigrants with skills used in finding employment, such as resume writing. Clinicians and case managers can assist in the application for low-cost bus fares and free cell phones based on psychological disabilities. These are services of which immigrants may not be aware and that make the transition to the USA less stressful. Affordable housing is also an issue, especially in heavily populated areas of the country, such as the San Francisco Bay area. Providing resources and helping immigrants with affordable housing applications, often in an unfamiliar language, can be crucial. Along with these resettlement agencies, CST has close relationships with charitable organizations such as the Second Harvest Food Bank. CST staff helps immigrants obtain weekly food stipends, which helps reduce stress regarding their basic needs. Every year, CST seeks dozens of donated bicycles which are specifically purposed for clients within the program.

Immigrant youth may be in an educational transition, wherein they have graduated from high school in their home country but are seeking higher education in the USA. It may be necessary to help individuals become familiar with the college application process and what is expected of an 18-year-old applicant. In general, it may be necessary to normalize individuals' place in society as expectations in one country for an 18-year-old may be very different in another country. These resources and foci of treatment do not fall within traditional mental health care and are all examples of assistance that makes the immigration and acculturation process less anxiety provoking and overwhelming.

Case Study

Seventeen-year-old "Amin" immigrated from Iran 9 months prior to the initial intake. He came to the USA seeking more educational opportunities and suffered from symptoms of depression and anxiety resulting from the resettlement process. He was particularly concerned about his education, place in society, and his career. Part of treatment with "Amin" was normalizing his expectations as a college student and providing appropriate resources so that he may better understand how the education system works and how different types of education lead to different types of careers. While he was concerned that he did not have the same financial situation as his peers, he slowly seemed to appreciate that his goals were long term. The therapist encouraged the client to make connections with his peers. In turn, he recognized that his mood increased with greater social connections.

Many of the patients utilizing these services suffer from major mental health disorders, most typically post-traumatic stress disorder. Therefore, along with the case managers, social workers, counselors, psychologists, and psychiatrists play an important role in providing mental health treatment to these individuals while they are trying to navigate problems with housing, food, and immigration law. Furthermore, these services are not provided in a vacuum. Psychotherapists help clients navigate the immigration process, and case managers provide emotional support. Knowledge of immigration law, housing opportunities, and food services is important to administering treatment in CST's holistic approach. Adding to this complicated form of treatment may be the need for a primary care physician to assist with various medical conditions. A case manager and/or mental health clinician often assist in obtaining one. For a detailed explanation of a refugee program modeled at CST, see Nazzal et al. [44].

As the client's cognitive space is freed with the amelioration of these more basic worries, room becomes open for emotional processing and more intensive therapy. Furthermore, assisting clients with these basic needs often improves mental health. Mental health treatment within this context is challenging. These systems are complicated and often unclear. It is important that mental health workers within these contexts are able to understand and navigate such systems (see Table 1 for general overview).

Table 1 Categories of youth immigration and the corresponding possible system navigation needs; these needs are not exhaustive

Designation	Possible system navigation needs (above and beyond basic needs such as food and shelter)
Voluntary immigration	Employment, immigration process, connection with religious/cultural community, mental health services
Refugee	Employment, connection with religious/cultural community, mental health services
Child trafficked	Employment, mental health services, criminal attorney, immigration process, primary care physician
Political asylum	Employment, mental health services, immigration process, primary care physician

Trauma and Grief

The immigration to a new country, even voluntarily, offers many opportunities for a child to become psychologically traumatized. Traumatizing experiences such as war, persecution, and economic disadvantage may have led to migration, and the process of leaving the home country may have involved the act of hiding, capture, mistreatment, exploitation, dangerous terrain, bigotry, and marginalization in an intermediate country [45, 46]. The process is enormously stressful, and anxiety and depression are commonly present [47]. Adjustment to a new life in a new country requires flexibility and resilience. Oftentimes, this flexibility and resilience is a matter of understanding what opportunities are available for refugees, making the work with the youth refugee population so unique. Mental health counselors and case managers have the ability to provide youth with resources mentioned above, which, in turn, ameliorates stress and allows for emotional and cognitive processing of their past and current environment.

Regardless of the manner of their arrival, all immigrants have sustained substantial losses, and those losses must be grieved. For voluntary immigrants, that grieving is somewhat tempered by the attainment of a goal and hopefully the benefits that derive from it. Mental health counselors and case managers, because they understand developmentally appropriate goals for living in the USA (e.g., graduating high school, working a summer job, obtaining a driver's license), can help these youth understand what is available to them and how to attain it. They are able to point youth toward the direction of certain communities that foster a sense of gaining benefits from society through school, work, family, religion, etc.

Those who arrive as the result of their involuntary displacement have little solace for their losses, which makes the task of grieving more difficult. The degree of flexibility and personal strengths strongly affects the immigrant's ability to adjust to their new life: these are qualities that are more associated with youth. Typically, younger people are much better able to accommodate to their new life circumstances and gradually construct a new life which compensates them, to some degree, for their losses [48]. Again, the unique opportunity to work with refugee youth allows mental health counselors and case managers to work toward emotional and cognitive processing of these losses while slowly introducing ways that youth can integrate themselves into their diaspora, American culture, or both. This is another example where providing traditional psychotherapy and case management services may play an integral role in providing optimal mental health treatment.

Acculturation Versus Preservation

The concepts of marginalization, separation, integration, and assimilation are separate forms or strategies of acculturation defined and introduced by John Berry [48] (Table 2). Marginalization is externally imposed by the dominant society, in which the immigrant community is isolated and disadvantaged [48]. Separation is self-imposed, wherein the immigrant community seeks to retain the customs and culture of their home country within their new circumstances [48]. Integration is the

Table 2 John Berry's [48] acculturative processes

Marginalization	Externally imposed by the dominant society; the immigrant community is isolated and disadvantaged
Separation	Self-imposed; immigrants within their respective communities seek to retain the customs and culture of their home country within their new circumstances
Integration	The selection of the old combined with the selection of the new customs and culture
Assimilation	Complete acceptance and identification with the dominant culture

selection of the old combined with the selection of the new customs and culture [48]. Assimilation is the complete acceptance and identification with the dominant culture [48]. Clinicians should be familiar with all of these concepts as they may encounter a number of them, even within a family system. Depending on which acculturative process a youth endorses, different social systems may be indicated. For instance, if a refugee youth endorses separation as the primary acculturative process, guiding her toward a church that places equal value in the US culture and premigration culture may be harmful to the therapeutic process, as the youth may understand this as the therapist or case manager not understanding her needs. Conversely, introducing a progressive youth who endorses the assimilation process to a church who endorses more traditional values may have the same effect.

Adults voluntarily immigrating to the USA generally attain integration as their form of acculturation. While valuing and sometimes idealizing their new country, their enthusiasm often dims with the realities of life in the USA and moves into a phase of disillusionment [49]. With time that phase may move into an acceptance of the disappointing realities. Ultimately and ideally, they are able to retain the best of the old while adopting the best of the new, finding their identity in their new country through integration.

Children, adolescents in particular, typically seek to become assimilated. They may go to extremes in their process of adaptation, wanting to fully adopt their new circumstances and culture, and reject all the dress, customs, and even language that their parents hope to honor and retain, at least in part [49, 50]. These conflicting goals often create friction between parents and their children and consequent stress for both [51]. It is common for refugees and asylum seekers who have been forced to leave their home country to adjust through isolation, that is, to seek out other members of the ethnic, religious, and/or linguistic community and operate as much as possible within that group. Typically traumatized by their experiences of persecution, they may have difficulty learning the new language and culture. With disorders such as PTSD, being able to learn new information may not be possible [52] which affects language acquisition. Without the ability to learn a new language, cultural isolation is more likely to occur and to be maintained. Like the voluntary immigrant children, refugee children who are younger seek assimilation, wanting to adopt the language, dress, and customs of their peers. Older children may be more influenced by their parents' isolation and seek to integrate the customs of their originating country with those of their new home.

Part of the parents' desire for their children to limit their adoption of the new culture is their own dream of someday returning "home" to their country of origin if changes occur in the political or social circumstances that led to their persecution. For most, however, it remains an unfulfilled dream. Even after becoming eligible for citizenship, many refugees fail to apply for it. Avoidance of further contact with the Immigration and Customs Enforcement, unfamiliarity with procedures, and resistance to taking a final step toward the loss of their home (from their perspective) all can play a part [53].

Children as Cultural Brokers

Case Study

While interpreting for her father being examined to determine if he was eligible for a citizenship interview waiver, which involves a psychological or medical professional attesting to his inability to learn English or civics due to a disability, 15-year-old "Anna" learned he'd been imprisoned and tortured for 2 years in their home country. Her father had failed to attend rallies and other displays of support for the Ethiopian government and was assumed to support its opposition. Suspension, beatings, exposure to extreme heat, and being forced to witness the torture and execution of others were among the various forms of torture to which he had been subjected. She was horrified and shocked at this revelation: as a child, she had been told he was on an extended business trip.

As described in Chapter 8, "Family Factors: Immigrant Families and Intergenerational Considerations," the children of immigrants are often placed into a position of being a buffer, or cultural broker, for their parents and their new culture. While their parents expect them to uphold the values and customs of their home country, they also need their children's understanding of the new culture, as well as their ability to speak and read English, to help them navigate the immigration and social service agencies with which they are compelled to interact. Children often learn a new language faster than their parents, and as such parents often rely on them to help ease the transition [54, 55]. Language brokering is defined as when youth with no formal training translate and interpret between two or more linguistically different parties [56–58]. Previous research has suggested that brokering begins within 1–5 years of arrival [54].

Language brokering occurs most frequently for parents but also includes other relatives, neighbors, and individuals within the community [55, 56]. The task of brokering occurs in a broad number of situations, including schools, banks, doctors' offices, and public domains. When doing so, the children must recognize the needs of others and understand how their skills can benefit others [56]. As children gain more linguistic ability and grasp of the host language, brokering may increase [56]. The use of children as interpreters is widely accepted in immigrant communities, but has faced criticism due to perceived disadvantages [54]. The debate regarding whether language brokering is an advantage or a disadvantage for children is examined in multiple studies.

Some research suggests that parental respect and attachment increase in accordance with language brokering, while others suggest that role reversal occurs, in turn undermining parental authority [54, 56]. Switching back and forth between the subservient child and the knowledgeable teacher, a child is often frustrated by her/his parents' seeming inability to learn basic concepts and their resistance to foreign ideas. This can be stressful on both sides. The accuracy of translated information may be questionable, and the information itself may negatively affect the mental health of child interpreters [54, 55]. For instance, a child like "Anna" in the case example above may become vicariously traumatized if he or she translates a parent's traumatic events and/or medical information [54]. In fact, lawmakers have entered the debate with a 2002 California bill that prohibits children from translating information in medical and legal situations [54].

For those that begin brokering at a young age, brokering is seen as normative and a practical way to contribute to the family [57]. Another benefit is it has also been found to foster an interest in culture and heritage that would otherwise be lost [55, 56]. Furthermore, in translating for parents, children are afforded the opportunity to practice their language [55]. Language abilities may be acquired at a faster rate with a higher vocabulary due to the increased exposure in diverse settings [54]. Children also have feelings of pride in their language abilities as well as their role in helping others in their family [55].

Current research suggests that Western mentality influences the thoughts of whether brokering is beneficial or detrimental to youth and instead should be looked at within an independent and interdependent frame of reference [57]. The feelings and thoughts associated with the act of brokering, more than the act of brokering per se, influence whether it is an advantage or disadvantage [58]. This is dependent on whether the act of brokering results in feelings of burden or empowerment [55]. Language brokering requires further study in light of the complex processes and multifaceted results that have been found.

Conclusion

Multiple governmental entities are in place to allow for the safe immigration of thousands of children into the USA every year. There are multiple avenues by which children come to the USA, seeking political asylum being one of them. Once here, it is often up to the community and nonprofit organizations to help their families gain access to life's basic needs. Refugees and other children seeking political asylum bring with them a history that may or not be categorized as traumatizing [49].

If youth are traumatized, the adjustment period is qualitatively different due to both the country from which they came and the steps it will take to gain permanent legal status in the USA. Navigating these systems can be difficult and overwhelming for both the child and mental health professionals [49]. Flexibility is essential.

Youth are in a unique position to be a conduit of resilience for the entire family. Youth are often left powerless and largely dependent on their parents by governmental influences and influences from their home countries. However, they have the flexibility needed to navigate these barriers toward adjustment [3]. Because of this, however, they may face enormous pressures from their parents to be even more successful than them. After all, their parents have often moved to benefit their children [59]. Understanding the cultural demands of the immigrant youth experience and supporting this experience through validation and empathy can go a long way toward a meaningful adjustment period. Social workers, counselors, psychologists, and psychiatrists all can play an important role in helping a child navigate these systems.

References

1. Dow HD. An overview of stressors faced by immigrants and refugees: a guide for mental health practitioners. Home Health Care Manag Pract. 2011;23(3):210–7.
2. Tribe R. Mental health of refugees and asylum-seekers. Adv Psychiatr Treat. 2002;8(4):240–7.
3. Masten A. Ordinary magic: resilience processes in development. Am Psychol. 2001;56(3): 227–38.
4. Jablensky A, Marsella AJ, Ekblad S, Jansson B, Levi L, Borneman T. Refugee mental health and well-being: conclusions and recommendations. In: Marsella AJ, Borneman T, Ekblad S, Orley J, editors. Amidst peril and pain. The mental health and well-being of the world's refugees. Washington, DC: American Psychological Association; 1994. p. 327–39.
5. UNHCR. Asylum-seekers; 2015. Retrieved from http://www.unhcr.org/pages/49c3646c137. html
6. UN General Assembly, Draft Convention relating to the Status of Refugees, 14 December 1950, A/RES/429. Retrieved from http://www.refworld.org/docid/3b00f08a27.html
7. USCIS. Refugees; 2015. Retrieved from http://www.uscis.gov/humanitarian/refugees-asylum/ refugees
8. Fazel M, Reed R, Tyrer R. Treating forcibly displaced young people: global challenges in mental health care. In: Patel S, Reicherter D, editors. Psychotherapy for immigrant youth. New York: Springer; 2015.
9. UNHCR. Global report: North America and the Caribbean subregional overview; 2009. Retrieved from http://www.unhcr.org/4c08f28f9.html
10. Office of Immigration Statistics. 2013 yearbook of immigration statistics; 2014. Retrieved from http://www.dhs.gov/sites/default/files/publications/ois_yb_2013_0.pdf
11. Pyszczynski T, Kesebir P. Anxiety buffer disruption theory: a terror management account of posttraumatic stress disorder. Anxiety Stress Coping. 2011;24(1):3–26.
12. Janoff-Bulman R. Assumptive worlds and the stress of traumatic events: applications of the schema construct. Soc Cogn. 1989;7:113–36.
13. Janoff-Bulman R. Shattered assumptions: towards a new psychology of trauma. New York: Free Press; 1992.
14. Abdollahi A, Pyszczynski T, Maxfield M, Luszczynska A. Posttraumatic stress reactions as a disruption in anxiety-buffer functioning: dissociation and responses to mortality salience as predictors of severity of posttraumatic symptoms. Psychol Trauma. 2011;3(4):329.

15. Greenberg J, Pyszczynski T, Solomon S. The causes and consequences of a need for self-esteem: a terror management theory. In: Baumeister RF, editor. Public self and private self. New York: Springer; 1986. p. 189–212.

16. Chatard A, Pyszczynski T, Arndt J, Selimbegović L, Konan PN, Van der Linden M. Extent of trauma exposure and PTSD symptom severity as predictors of anxiety-buffer functioning. Psychol Trauma. 2012;4(1):47.

17. Edmondson D, Chaudoir SR, Mills MA, Park CL, Holub J, Bartkowiak JM. From shattered assumptions to weakened worldviews: trauma symptoms signal anxiety buffer disruption. J Loss Trauma. 2011;16(4):358–85.

18. Kesebir P, Luszczynska A, Pyszczynski T, Benight C. Posttraumatic stress disorder involves disrupted anxiety-buffer mechanisms. J Soc Clin Psychol. 2011;30(8):819–41. doi:10.1521/jscp.2011.30.8.819.

19. Pyszczynski T, Greenberg J, Solomon S, Arndt J, Schimel J. Why do people need self-esteem? A theoretical and empirical review. Psychol Bull. 2004;130(3):435–68.

20. USCIS. Asylum; 2015. Retrieved from http://www.uscis.gov/humanitarian/refugees-asylum/asylum

21. UNHCR. Handbook and guidelines on procedures and criteria for determining refugee status; 2011. Retrieved from http://www.unhcr.org/3d58e13b4.html

22. USCIS. I-589 Application for asylum and withholding of removal; 2015. Retrieved from http://www.uscis.gov/sites/default/files/files/form/i-589.pdf

23. Cox P. Issues in safeguarding refugee and asylum-seeking children and young people: research and practice. Child Abuse Rev. 2011;20(5):341–60. doi:10.1002/car.1200.

24. NOLO. When an asylee or refugee can apply for U.S. citizenship; 2015. Retrieved from http://www.nolo.com/legal-encyclopedia/when-asylee-refugee-can-apply-us-citizenship.html

25. United States Department of Justice. Asylum statistics; 2014. Retrieved from http://www.justice.gov/sites/default/files/eoir/legacy/2014/04/16/FY2009-FY2013AsylumStatisticsbyNationality.pdf

26. USCIS. Questions and answers: appeals and motions; 2015. http://www.uscis.gov/forms/questions-and-answers-appeals-and-motions

27. Amnesty International. US: Catch-22 for Asylum Seekers; 2013. https://www.hrw.org/news/2013/11/12/us-catch-22-asylum-seekers

28. USCIS. Minor children applying for asylum by themselves; 2015. http://www.uscis.gov/humanitarian/refugees-asylum/asylum/minor-children-applying-asylum-themselves

29. Van Selm J. Public-private partnerships in refugee resettlement: Europe and the US. J Int Migr Integr. 2003;4(2):157–75.

30. Stein BN. The experience of being a refugee: insights from the research literature. In: Williams CL, Westermeyer J, editors. Refugee mental health in resettlement countries. Washington, DC: Hemisphere; 1986. p. 5–23.

31. Fix M, Zimmermann W, Passel J. The integration of immigrant families in the United States. Washington, DC: Urban Institute; 2001.

32. Miller KE, Rasmussen A. War exposure, daily stressors, and mental health in conflict and post-conflict settings: bridging the divide between trauma-focused and psychosocial frameworks. Soc Sci Med. 2010;70(1):7–16.

33. H.R. Res. 613, 106th Congress, 114 Cong. Rec. 3244 (2000) (enacted).

34. United States Department of State. Trafficking in persons report; 2004. Retrieved from http://www.state.gov/j/tip/rls/tiprpt/2004/34021.htm

35. National Human Trafficking Resource Center. T visa and the trauma exception; 2015. Retrieved from http://traffickingresourcecenter.org/resources/t-visa-and-trauma-exception

36. Barnett ED. Infectious disease screening for refugees resettled in the United States. Clin Infect Dis. 2004;39(6):833–41.

37. Cecchet SJ, Thoburn J. The psychological experience of child and adolescent sex trafficking in the United States: trauma and resilience in survivors. Psychol Trauma. 2014;6(5):482–93. doi:10.1037/a0035763.

38. Ijadi-Maghsoodi R, Todd EJ, Bath EJ. Commercial sexual exploitation of children and the role of the child psychiatrist. J Am Acad Child Adolesc Psychiatry. 2014;53(8):825–9. doi:10.1016/j.jaac.2014.05.005.

39. Oppedal B, Idsoe T. The role of social support in the acculturation and mental health of unaccompanied minor asylum seekers. Scand J Psychol. 2015;56(2):203–11. doi:10.1111/sjop.12194.
40. Seugling CJ. Toward a comprehensive response to the transnational migration of unaccompanied minors in the United States. Vand J Transnat'l L. 2004;37(3):861–95.
41. Martinez LM. Dreams deferred: the impact of legal reforms on undocumented Latino youth. Am Behav Sci. 2014;58(14):1873–90. doi:10.1177/0002764214550289.
42. Lorentzen L, Gonzalez J, Chun K, Do I. Religion at the corner of bliss and nirvana: politics, identity and faith in new migrant communities. Durham: Duke University Press; 2009.
43. Donnelly TT, Hwang JJ, Este D, Ewashen C, Adair C, Clinton M. If I was going to kill myself, I wouldn't be calling you. I am asking for help: Challenges influencing immigrant and refugee women's mental health. Issues Ment Health Nurs. 2011;32(5):279–90. doi:10.3109/01612840 .2010.550383.
44. Nazzal KH, Forghany M, Geevarughese MC, Mahmoodi V, Wong J. An innovative community-oriented approach to prevention and early intervention with refugees in the United States. Psychol Serv. 2014;11(4):477.
45. Infante C, Idrovo AJ, Sánchez-Domínguez MS, Vinhas S, González-Vázquez T. Violence committed against migrants in transit: experiences on the northern Mexican border. J Immigr Minor Health. 2012;14(3):449–59.
46. Perreira KM, Ornelas IJ. The physical and psychological well-being of immigrant children. Futur Child. 2011;21(1):195–218.
47. Pumariega AJ, Rothe E, Pumariega JB. Mental health of immigrants and refugees. Commun Ment Health J. 2005;41(5):581–97.
48. Berry JW. Immigration, acculturation, and adaptation. Appl Psychol. 1997;46(1):10.
49. Alvarez M. The experience of migration: a relational approach in therapy. J Fem Fam Ther. 1999;11(1):1–29. doi:10.1300/J086v11n01_01.
50. Igoa C. The inner world of the immigrant child. New York: St. Martin's Press; 1995.
51. Castillo LG, Zahn MP, Cano MA. Predictors of familial acculturative stress in Asian American College students. J Coll Couns. 2012;15:52–64.
52. Jenkins MA, Langlais PJ, Delis D, Cohen R. Learning and memory in rape victims with post-traumatic stress disorder. Am J Psychiatr. 1998;155(2):278–9.
53. Bloemraad I. Becoming a citizen in the United States and Canada: structured mobilization and immigrant political incorporation. Soc Forces. 2006;85(2):667–95.
54. Morales A, Hanson WE. Language brokering: an integrative review of the literature. Hisp J Behav Sci. 2005;27(4):471–503. doi:10.1177/0739986305281333.
55. Weisskirch RS. Family relationships, self-esteem, and self-efficacy among language brokering Mexican American emerging adults. J Child Fam Stud. 2013;22(8):1147–55. doi:10.1007/ s10826-012-9678-x.
56. Dorner LM, Orellana MF, Jiménez R. 'It's one of those things that you do to help the family': Language brokering and the development of immigrant adolescents. J Adolesc Res. 2008;23(5):515–43. doi:10.1177/0743558408317563.
57. Kam JA. The effects of language brokering frequency and feelings on Mexican-heritage youth's mental health and risky behaviors. J Commun. 2011;61(3):455–75. doi:10.1111/j.1460-2466.2011.01552.x.
58. Kam JA, Lazarevic V. The stressful (and not so stressful) nature of language brokering: identifying when brokering functions as a cultural stressor for Latino immigrant children in early adolescence. J Youth Adolesc. 2014;43(12):1994–2011. doi:10.1007/s10964-013-0061-z.
59. Roubeni S, De Haene L, Keatley E, Shah N, Rasmussen A. 'If we can't do it, our children will do it one day': a qualitative study of West African immigrant parents' losses and educational aspirations for their children. Am Educ Res J. 2015;52(2):275–305. doi:10.3102/ 0002831215574576.

Erratum to: Psychotherapy for Immigrant Youth

Sita G. Patel and Daryn Reicherter

© Springer International Publishing Switzerland 2016
S. Patel, D. Reicherter (eds.), *Psychotherapy for Immigrant Youth*,
DOI 10.1007/978-3-319-24693-2

DOI 10.1007/978-3-319-24693-2_10

Erratum to:

The middle initial G has to be added to Sita Patel. The name should read Sita G. Patel in title page, copyright page, cover and in about the editors.

Introduction:

Page vii- line 29- The middle initial E. has to be removed from Erynn E. Macciomei. The name should read Erynn Macciomei

Page vii- line 29- The middle initial G has to be added to Sita Patel. The name should read Sita G. Patel

Page viii- line 32- A comma has to be added between the names James Livingston and Marilee Ruebsamen.

The updated online version of the original book can be found under
http://dx.doi.org/10.1007/978-3-319-24693-2

Sita Patel
Palo Alto University
Palo Alto, CA, USA

Daryn Reicherter, MD
Stanford University School of Medicine
Palo Alto, CA, USA

© Springer International Publishing Switzerland 2016
S. Patel, D. Reicherter (eds.), *Psychotherapy for Immigrant Youth*,
DOI 10.1007/978-3-319-24693-2_10

Page viii- line 33- A suffix II has to be added to David E. Reed and should read as David E. Reed II

Page viii- line 32/33 The order of authors has to changed to: David E. Reed II, Marilee Ruebsamen, James Livingston, and Fazia Eltareb.

Page ix- line 6- The middle initial G has to be added to Sita Patel. The name should read Sita G. Patel

Contents:

Page xiii- line 5- The middle initial G has to be added to Sita Patel. The name should read Sita G. Patel

Page xiii- line 11/12- The order of authors has to changed to: Micaela A. Thordarson, Marisa Keller, Paul J. Sullivan, Sandra Trafalis, and Robert D. Friedberg

Page xiv- line 10- A suffix II has to be added to David E. Reed and should read as David E. Reed II

Page xiv- line 10- The spelling for name Ruebsamen is wrong. It must be changed to "Ruebsamen"

Contributors

Page xv- line 1- The designation is missing. The name should be Rania Awaad, M.D.

Page xv- line 4- The designation is missing. The name should be Guadalupe Bacio, Ph.D.

Page xv- line 7- The name must be updated to Eduardo Bunge, Ph.D.

Page xv- line 12- The designation is missing. The name should be Victor Carrion, M.D.

Page xv- line 15- The designation is missing. The name should be Diana Capous, M.A.

Page xv- line 18- The designation is missing. The name should be Margareth Del Cid, M.A.

Page xv- line 21- The designation is missing. The name should be Benjamin Dickter, M.A.

Page xv- line 26- The designation is missing. The name should be Fazia Eltareb, M.S.

Page xv- line 34- The name must be updated to Megan K. Jones, B.S.

Page xv- line 36- The designation is missing. The name should be Linda Juang, Ph.D.

Page xv- line 38- The designation is missing. The name should be Marisa Keller, M.S.

Page xvi- line 1- The designation is missing. The name should be Maryam Kia-Keating, Ph.D.

Page xvi- line 5- The designation is missing. The name should be HilitKletter, Ph.D.

Page xvi- line 8- The designation is missing. The name should be James Livingston, Ph.D.

Page xvi- line 11- The designation is missing. The name should be Erynn Macciomei, M.S.

Page xvi- line 17- The designation is missing. The name should be Yasmin Owusu, M.D.

Page xvi- line 20- The designation is missing. The name should be Rosaura Perales, B.A.

Page xvi- line 22- A suffix II has to be added to David E. Reed and should read as David E. Reed II

Page xvi- line 24- Add a middle initial and update credentials as Ruth V. Reed, MB BChir MRCPCH, MRCPsych

Page xvi- line 24- Kindly change affiliation to Oxford Health NHS Foundation Trust, Warneford Hospital, Oxford, UK

Page xvi- line 27- Delete entry for Daryn Reicherter on the Contributor list

Page xvi- line 30- The designation is missing. The name should be John P. Rettger, Ph.D.

Page xvi- line 33- The designation is missing. The name should be Marilee Ruebsamen, Ph.D. (correct spelling and credential)

Page xvi- line 35- The designation is missing. The name should be Anna Staudenmeyer, M.S.

Page xvi- line 38- The designation is missing. The name should be Andrea Spear, M.A.

Page xvi- line 40- The designation is missing. The name should be Paul J. Sullivan, M.S.

Page xvi- line 43- The designation is missing. The name should be Micaela J. Thordarson, M.S.

Page xvi- line 46- The designation is missing. The name should be Sandra Trafalis, Ph.D.

Page xvi- line 49- The designation is missing. The name should be Rebecca Tyrer, B.Sc., M.Res.

Chapter 1

Page 3- Line 3- The middle initial G has to be added to Sita Patel. The name should read Sita G. Patel

Page 3- In the copyright footnote at the end of EACH chapter please add the middle initial G. to S. Patel and make it as S.G. Patel

Chapter 2

Page 27- The authors order should be: Micaela A. Thordarson, Marisa Keller, Paul J. Sullivan, Sandra Trafalis, and Robert D. Friedberg

Chapter 9- Reed, Livingston

Please change all headers for this chapter to D. E. Reed II et al.

Page 167- chapter author name corrections and footnote

A suffix II has to be added to David E. Reed and should read as David E. Reed II

Please correct spelling from Reubsamen to Ruebsamen

Cultural Perspectives in the Context of Western Psychological Mind-sets: The Need for Cultural Sensitivity in the Mental Health of Immigrant Youth

Rania Awaad and Daryn Reicherter

Abstract

Before psychotherapeutic interventions for *immigrant youth* are considered, a context must be examined in which psychological/psychiatric diagnoses and treatment strategies are understood. In this chapter, we discuss the imperative of incorporating cultural context in psychotherapy, beginning with a definition and examination of cross-cultural psychiatry. We then provide an analysis of the Western narrative of the history of psychology and psychiatry as disciplines and refocus to reveal the antecedence of parallel, non-Western developments in psychology. Further, we describe the insular nature of modern Western psychological research and the necessity of diversifying the samples studied or qualifying research as relevant to the particular communities who participated in the studies. We then move on to evaluate the vocabulary used by different cultures and explain why the recently developed Western lexicon does not function as a universal language given its incongruence with many beliefs of non-Western cultures. A discussion of religion and psychology is followed by an exploration of the controversial Universalism-Cultural Relativism debate, with particular emphasis placed on the flashpoint of culture-bound syndromes.

Keywords

Cultural sensitivity • Immigrant • Cross cultural • Culture-bound syndrome • Spirituality

R. Awaad (✉) • D. Reicherter
Department of Psychiatry and Behavioral Sciences, Stanford University School of Medicine, Stanford, CA, USA
e-mail: rawaad@stanford.edu

Cultural Sensitivity in the Mental Health of Immigrants

The book, "*Psychotherapy for Immigrant Youth*," was an accumulation of updated, evidence-based information about how best to approach the delivery of psychotherapy for this vulnerable population. The sections throughout the book elaborated different mental health treatment approaches for the broad population category of *immigrant youth*. But some assumptions about psychopathology and its treatments are culturally relative. This appendix, "Cultural Perspectives in the Context of Western Psychological Mind-sets: The Need for Cultural Sensitivity in the Mental Health of Immigrant Youth," points out the notion that cultural context must be considered whenever examining the utility or applicability of Western mental health treatment on non-Western populations. Given the wide spectrum of non-Western traditions and understandings in regard to human psychological experience, immigrant youth and their families may have very different responses to intervention by Western trained mental health professionals. Cultural understanding is an essential root in the approach to immigrant mental health and especially for the consideration of psychotherapy for immigrant youth.

Culture and Mental Health

"Cross-cultural" or "Intercultural" Psychiatry is becoming a norm rather than the exception given the United States' changing demographics and immigrations throughout the world. It is more common now than ever before that a mental health professional will work with a person of a different cultural background. For the purposes of this chapter, we can define "intercultural" mental health treatment as a clinical treatment situation wherein the identified patient is of one cultural background and the clinician is of another. For example, this scenario can be achieved when a Caucasian psychiatrist from Kansas works clinically with a Hmong refugee family from Laos: both clinician and client having very different cultural backgrounds and concepts about psychological norms, psychological pathology, and appropriate interventions for psychology. But intercultural mental health treatment can also occur in the context of a psychologist identifying as culturally Vietnamese working with an English-speaking child born and raised in Australia: again, both clinician and client possibly having very different cultural backgrounds and concepts about psychological norms, psychological pathology, and appropriate interventions for psychology.

The necessary consideration of culture in conceptualizing psychology and its pathologies is becoming more and more apparent as practitioners find failure with the current diagnostic and treatment processes in regard to effectiveness. While the American Diagnostic and Statistical Manual of Mental Disorders (DSM) and other conventions for evaluating and assessing diagnoses make attempts to capture the essence of a mental health disorder, it may be difficult to interpret symptoms through the filter of language and cultural bias. Non-Western models for explaining psychological symptoms or states or categorizing disorder diagnosis can be very different from standard Western convention.

Once clinical diagnosis is conceptualized, intervention may be very difficult to apply, given the very different notions about what interventions apply from a cultural standpoint. There may be as many biases around what intervention to use for a psychological/psychiatric problem as there are cultures. Even when mental health providers look to evidence-based literature for guidance, they must weigh the amount to which studies incorporate cultural diversity before determining the legitimacy of literature when applied to specific intercultural situations.

Cultural sensitivity, therefore, must become new standard for thinking about the use of different modalities of psychotherapeutic intervention in the modern climate of diversity. There is a role for psychotherapy in intercultural mental health treatment. But it is open to scrutiny and examination. It is more complicated than would simply allow for the application of non-culturally specific, evidence-based Western psychotherapy models without completely incorporating cultural sensitivity.

A History of the Western Model of Psychology

Western psychological practice has been greatly ethnocentric at least in part due to its claim to the origins of psychological science. The majority of Western anthologies on the history of psychology do not acknowledge other cultural views of psychology outside of Europe and rarely attempt to trace back psychology's historic origins beyond the Greeks and Romans [1–4]. Widely referenced histories of Western psychology imply that, until the research and writings of German psychologists Gustov Fechner and Wilhelm Wudnt in the late 1800s, psychology was not considered a discipline and therefore did not exist as psychology [5]. Early movements in psychology in the Victorian Age may define the early history of the discipline of Western psychology for some historians, but there is a rich tradition in the art and science of psychology in the West and in other traditions that predates this.

Rich, ancient traditions filled with psychological thought can be found in Chinese and Indian writings that predate the Greeks. The core tenants of many Eastern religious movements, like Buddhism, center on human psychological experience and have developed for millennia. The unprecedented advancements in medicine and psychology made during the Islamic Golden Era is another example of an early and parallel movement toward understanding psychology often unmentioned in the historical accounts of the discipline of psychology [6].

When considering the DSM 5 and American-based evidence-based literature on mental health interventions, it should be noted that Americans comprise less than 5 % of the world's population [7]. Thus, using Western ideals and standards as the lens through which we view psychology can result in an understanding of psychology that is incomplete and that can neither adequately represent nor serve all populations. Instead, objective historical understanding of psychological theory and practice as a human, cross-cultural endeavor is necessary as is the development of a more culturally inclusive and astute body of psychological theory and practice (Table 1).

Table 1 Problems with exclusive use of Euro-American psychology

Attributes of Euro-American psychology	Resulting problems
Largely originated in the late 1800s with the writings of Fechner and Wudnt	Ignores the rich history of Eastern psychological science
Research subjects primarily white, middle class	Research findings inapplicable to a great majority of people in need of treatment
Born in a society that stigmatizes people with mental illnesses	Largely does not reserve sympathy or reverence for the mentally ill, as is often done in Eastern traditions
Suggests religion is a consequence of psychopathology	Incongruous with many cultures that highly value religion

Important Cultural Aspects in the Experience of Psychology

The tendency in Western academic psychology to assume a universalistic cultural context has led to a diminished attention to the importance of Non-Western cultural considerations in psychology. This tendency has also led to skewed population sampling in research participants and bias in formulation of research questions. Jared Diamond notes that most psychological studies are done by white, middle-class researchers with subjects who are white and middle class [8]. Other critics have charged that the default and accepted understanding of the cultural context for human development is homogeneous [9]. That is to say that culture is based on a set standard of values and expectations primarily held by white, middle-class populations. For example, when children are referenced in published psychological research, they typically refer to white children [10] and women generally refer to white women [11]. Researchers only define populations' ethnicities when they refer to non-caucasians. Consequently, psychological research has adopted stances that are geared to treat middle-class, European-American research populations as the default subject of research and, consequently, the default subject of the evidence we base clinical decisions on.

Arnett [7], in his article, "The Neglected 95 %: Why American Psychology Needs to be Less American," demonstrated through examining 20 years of research presented in psychology journals that 95 % of the psychological studies are undertaken by Americans about Americans. Yet, "theories and principles are developed that are mistakenly assumed to apply to human beings in general; they are assumed to be universal." Arnett also pointed out that so little research has been dedicated to determining how psychology is understood by the rest of the world. Thus, academic books used for university classes may be more aptly titled *Euro-American Developmental Psychology* or *Abnormal American Psychology* than *Developmental Psychology* or *Abnormal Psychology*. American textbooks on psychology are now bought and circulated in universities abroad, fueling, in part, the growing movement against American constructs of psychology and mental health [12].

Different Fundamental Assumptions on the Theory of "Mind"

A Western concept of mind in both youth and adults is not universally held. The Western view of cognition holds that all learning and psychological development takes place within the brain and involves thinking. Yet, looking at this concept from a non-Western perspective points to it being a cultural and ethnocentric psychological viewpoint rather than objective reality [13, 14]. Western science does not currently accept or acknowledge the existence of nonlocal consciousness as is understood in many Eastern philosophies. Furthermore, research in the field of psychiatry and neurobiology has posited that consciousness, apart from the mechanisms of the brain, does not exist [15]. The reductionist approach used in Western science is prone to reducing all understanding of the psyche to chemical processes occurring in the brain.

Language is an important cultural consideration in our understanding of psychology. For example, the concept of "cognition" is heavily influenced by the Western cultural view of "the mind." However, this is not a universally agreed upon understanding. Other cultures assign different characteristics and abilities to the psychological aspects of personhood.

Cross-linguistic research has shown that many cultures have a folk model of personhood or "mind" that consists of visible and invisible (psychological) aspects [16]. In the English-speaking West, the psychological aspect of personhood is closely related to the concept of "the mind" and has strongly influenced the modern view of cognition. Other traditions have very different starting points.

In the Korean language, the concept "maum" replaces the concept of "mind." "Maum" has no English counterpart, but is sometimes translated as "heart." The closest description of "maum" in the English language is the "seat of emotions, motivation, and goodness in a human being" [16]. Intellect and cognitive functions are captured by the Korean term "meli" (head). However, "maum" is clearly the counterpart to "mind" in terms of the psychological part of the person.

The Japanese have yet another concept for the invisible, psychological part of a person. In Japanese language, "Kokoro" is a "seat of emotion" and also "a source of culturally valued attention to, and empathy with, other people" [16]. In contrast to the Korean "maum," "kokoro" is not associated with will and motivation ("hara" which means belly serves this purpose in Japanese). However, "hara" is not associated with the psychological component of a person. In other words, Korean "maum" refers to motivation, Japanese "kokoro" refers to feelings, and the Western concept of the "mind" refers to thinking.

Russian languages use "dusa" as the counterpart to the psychological part of the person. "Dusa" is often translated as "soul," but also sometimes as "heart" or "mind." "Dusa" is associated with feelings, morality, and spirituality. The "dusa" is responsible for the ability to connect with other people. This meaning seems to resonate more with the Eastern conceptualization of the invisible, psychological aspects of a person than with the highly cognitive Western concept of the "mind" (Table 2).

Had Western cognitive psychology developed out of the Korean, Japanese, or Russian traditions, it is unlikely that the "mind" would have played such a crucial

Table 2 Personhood, as it is understood in a number of selected cultures

Culture	Definition of personhood
Western	One's identity is dominated by "the mind," which influences cognition and consciousness
Korean	"Maum" is the closest equivalent to "mind" in the West, but it also takes on the specific responsibilities of being in control of emotions, motivations, and goodness
Japanese	"Kokoro" contains one's emotions and sense of empathy, but does not include motivation, which is not typically associated with one's psychology
Russian	"Dusa" encompasses feelings, morality, spirituality, and empathy

role in the understanding of psychology. This possibility highlights the arbitrariness of how the psychological realm is currently carved out—what is believed to be objective reality is in fact heavily dependent on culture, language, and traditional origin.

Western Psychiatry and Spirituality

Spiritual and religious understandings of the psyche are an equally important cultural consideration and apply to psychology in youth and adults. At the end of the nineteenth century and beginning of the twentieth, French neurologist Jean Charcot (and later his star pupil, Sigmund Freud) linked religion with hysteria and neurosis [17]. Freud's opinions significantly contributed to the development of Western psychology and largely helped define the relationship between religion and psychiatry. It was not until the publication of the DSM 4 in 1994 that examples depicting religious persons as being mentally ill ceased [18].

For over a century, many Western clinicians have thought of the religious beliefs and practices of their patients as having a pathological basis, especially if the religion is non-Western. Recent research has challenged deeply entrenched stance held by Western psychology. In some cases, hallucinations may even be a life-enhancing experience: for example, hearing voices of ancestors or guardian angels and finding comfort in them, or seeing visions and finding inspiration or religious revelation in them [19].

Other studies have uncovered findings that suggest religion may be a protective factor as well as a resource to some patients that helps them to cope with the stresses in life, including those of their illness [17, 20]. Despite these robust findings, people with prominent psychotic symptoms in Western societies are likely to be stigmatized and isolated. By contrast, in many traditional societies these same people may be seen as visionaries and mystics and celebrated and sought out for their special insights and abilities.

This may have much to do with practice of conferring a shaman-like status to people who may project an aura of spirituality and religiosity due to high levels of paranormal and religious beliefs. The term "shaman" is generally used to refer to people with important roles in traditional societies such as healers, medicine men, seers, and sorcerers who are respected for abilities such as divining the weather, communing with the spirits, and placating the gods bringing about physical and psychological healing.

An interesting manifestation of spiritual and religious interpretation of mental illness can be exemplified in medieval Islamic society. In his significant study, *Majnun: The Madman in Medieval Islamic Society*, Michael W. Dols [21] argues that medieval Islamic civilization "permitted a much wider latitude to the interpretation of unusual behaviour than does modern Western society and much greater freedom to the disturbed, non-violent individual." Such societal acceptance allowed for a variety of states on the normality/abnormality scale and ensured that "the madman was accommodated by society, so that he was not a pariah, an outcast, or a scapegoat." Dols also pointed out that this flexibility explains the prevalent "methods of healing, modes of perceiving, and ways of protecting the insane" found in classical Islamic societies.

Some traditional societies welcomed the same people who may be marginalized in Western societies due to their history of treating religion as psychopathology. Thus, rather than being stigmatized and isolated, people with "madness," "psychosis," "schizophrenia" may be seen as gifted or blessed and may be accorded an important social role and potentially a high social status. Several investigators [22–25] have found that the outcome of schizophrenia is generally more favorable in traditional societies. This may be due in a large part to the conceptualization of mental disorders by people in traditional societies more as a part of life than as a sign of illness or failure. This essential shift in perception can be credited for enabling people with a mental disorder to retain an honorable place in the very midst of their societies.

In terms of clinical effectiveness with patients and patient families, these historical paths that lead to different understandings of psychology are important to understand in clinical diagnosis and treatment.

"Culture-Bound Syndromes"

Culturally specific syndromes provide another example to consider and criticize the universality of mental health diagnoses and intervention. The so-called *Culture-bound syndromes*, also known as *culture-specific disorders*, refer to mental illnesses or behavioral disturbances that are unique to, and are understandable only in the context of, a certain culture. Many examples of these were given in Western accounts of cross-cultural psychiatry. In the appendix of the DSM IV, 25 "Culture-bound syndromes" are described in a selectively inclusive glossary. In the appendix, many behavioral phenomena are described without contextualization in the cultural circumstance in which it is understood. According to the *Dictionary of Psychology*, culture-bound syndromes are patterns of behavior that do not fit accordingly into normal classifications of mental disorders. They "are entirely or mainly restricted to particular cultural groups" [40].

Culture-bound disorders came into Western psychiatric literature in the late nineteenth century, when Western physicians made reports of strange and "exotic" disorders they observed while working in Asia, Africa, and South America. They noticed that these disorders were different from the disorders found in Europe and North America. More than 50 culture-bound disorders have been reported in the clinical and research literature. However, only a few receive the most attention and are well known, such as *latah*, *amok*, and *susto*.

Every culture has its own and different "disorders" or (usually) maladaptive behavioral expressions that may or may not be modifications of the disorders found in the Western world that are said to be "universal"; this is why they are called culture-bound disorders (*Encyclopedia of Psychology*, 1994, p. 374). In theory, culture-bound syndromes are those "folk" illnesses in which alterations of behavior and experience figure prominently. In actuality, however, many are not syndromes at all. Instead, they are local ways of explaining any of a wide assortment of misfortunes [41].

Other more common disorders, even though they may share a biological or genetic substrate, are more likely to be shaped by social context, cultural norms, and developmental stage. Rutter and Nikapota argue in favor of integrating both a universal and relativistic view of psychopathology depending on the specific disorder. The extent to which the definitions of disorders or syndromes are universal across cultures or vary significantly across cultures is a matter to be determined by empirical inquiry that establishes the validity of the diagnostic criteria across cultures [42].

The combined relativistic and universalistic approach in diagnostic classificatory systems for psychopathology states that some disorders (i.e., autism, schizophrenia, fragile X syndrome, and other pervasive developmental disorders) are more likely to be universal in all cultures because they are mostly based on neural pathology [42].

But it is useful to fully examine a culture-bound syndrome beyond the phenomenology and understand the context in order to uncover the role that culture and worldview play in the expression of psychological events. For this exercise, consider the culture-bound syndrome seen in the East, koro. The DSM IV defines koro as "a term that refers to an episode of sudden and intense anxiety that the penis (or, in females, the vulva and nipples) will recede into the body and possibly cause death" (DSM IV).

Without context, this condition sounds like it might be thought of as an anxiety disorder or a body dysmorphic disorder. Reading about the phenomena as described in the DSM could also indicate that an individual with koro suffers from a psychotic belief, namely that the genitals are shrinking or that their shrinking could result in death. But the phenomenon occurs in a context of culture and worldview that makes the phenomena seem less like a psychotic delusion. The cultural beliefs that surround *koro* include ideas of sex physiology in the traditional Chinese medicine, which in fact links fatality with genital retraction. This is believed to be fact, not myth. In the ancient Chinese medical book *ZhongZang Jing*, retraction of the penis with distension of the abdomen was described as a certain sign of death. Yin and yang theory, widely appreciated in Asia, proposes that an unbalanced loss of the yang humor produces genital shrinkage. In Traditional Chinese medicine, frequent ejaculation is regarded as detrimental to health, as semen is considered to be related to a man's vital energy, and hence excessive depletion of semen may lead to illness or death. Some authors believe that the idea of death caused by the semen depletion resembles the idea of death caused by genital disappearance.

Some DSM IV disorders are listed in the body of the manual without explicit reference to cultural factors that might suggest the root of the illness. It has been debated whether eating disorders like *anorexia nervosa* have an intrinsic cultural element or even are (Western) culture-bound syndromes. In this case, the behavior may be steeped in the cultural link between thinness and beauty for females. In a culture without emphasis on thinness for beauty, the behaviors and beliefs of an anorexic may seem disorganized and bizarre. Other similar examples throughout the DSM are debated as to their cultural relevance.

When the cultural root or worldview is better understood, the mechanism for how a culture-bound syndrome comes to be understood by that culture becomes clearer. Also potential interventions or "cures" can be differentially prescribed when the underlying worldview is understood. Without the cultural understanding, the idiom of distress will not be understood and interventions cannot be well prescribed.

Universalism vs. Cultural Relativism

There is evidence that a person's cultural background colors every facet of their illness experience, from linguistic structure [26, 27] to the unique meaning of expressed emotion [28, 29]. Yet, there is little consensus on the extent to which these cultural factors influence psychiatric disorders causing them to differ on their core definitions and constellation of symptoms. This has led to controversy about the universality versus the relativity of psychiatric disorders or syndromes across cultural groups. In part, this controversy has been debated for many years due to the lack of biological markers, imprecise measurement, and ultimately the lack of a gold standard for validating most psychiatric conditions [30].

Research on culture and mental health has traditionally focused on one of two orientations. The first being the Universalist view that holds that similarities exist in mental disorders across all cultures, but the expression of these disorders varies from culture to culture. The other view is the Cultural Relativist approach. This view holds that some disorders are unique to a culture and may only be understood from a cultural perspective [31]. This relativistic point of view claims that culture shapes the individual's development and his/her biological and psychological unfolding to a substantial degree—thus calling for the need to integrate culture within the diagnostic classificatory system [32]. Otherwise, important cultural symptoms and syndromes unique to particular cultural settings result in a category fallacy or apparent homogeneity of disorders across cultures [33].

Thus, there exists a clear divide in the literature with adherents of biopsychological universalism interpreting mental illnesses as manifestations of universal human psychopathology, only influenced and modified by particular cultural factors [34–36]. On the other side, adherents of an ethnological cultural relativism purport these conditions as engendered or generated by aspects of a particular culture [37–39]. This divide has led to heated debates between both sides over the concept of "culture-bound syndromes." Though this debate may not find rest soon, these syndromes testify to the profound influence cultural factors exert on the human mind (Table 3).

Table 3 Universalism vs. cultural relativism

Universalism	Cultural relativism
Asserts that the same diseases exist across cultures, even if they are understood differently	Asserts that there exist certain diseases that only affect certain cultures or populations (culture-bound syndromes)
Suggests disorders are purely the result of biopsychological complications	Suggests disorders can be influenced by ethnology
Argues that diagnoses can be made independently of cultural considerations	Argues that diagnostic classifications must take culture into account
Can't be categorically proven due to linguistic disparities and the absence of a uniform, concrete, cross-cultural standard by which to evaluate the accuracy of diagnoses	

Cultural Sensitivity and Psychotherapy for Immigrant Youth

The Mayo Clinic web resource defines psychotherapy (for youth as well as adults) as follows: "Psychotherapy is a general term for treating mental health problems by talking with a psychiatrist, psychologist or other mental health provider." It continues, "During psychotherapy, you learn about your condition and your moods, feelings, thoughts and behaviors. Psychotherapy helps you learn how to take control of your life and respond to challenging situations with healthy coping skills. There are many specific types of psychotherapy, each with its own approach. The type of psychotherapy that's right for you depends on your individual situation. Psychotherapy is also known as talk therapy, counseling, psychosocial therapy or, simply, therapy."

In Western culture, psychotherapy has roots in a dynamic therapy developed in the Freudian tradition. This is an essential premise in understanding the way a Western trained mental health professional will approach a patient's psychology, their diagnosis, and treatment. In fact, Western language lexicons have been modified by the thoughts of Freud and his disciples. Terms like "ego" and "subconscious" have entered into the English language or have modified their meaning in the last 150 years as a result of the influence of psychodynamic psychology. The language is said to be "psychologized." This is not necessarily true of other languages. This is not to say that other languages lack the proper lexicon to describe psychological states. Only that they may not reflect a newly incorporated way of thinking about psychological terms, all of which come from one system of thought from one theory. The theory's validity is under question within its own cultural context and definitely not validated in other cultures.

The need for better cultural understanding of how psychotherapy might be incorporated into treatment plans from culture to culture is a subject of investigation for youth and adult patients. And the sensitivity to cultural norms around the manifestation, cause, and intervention in mental illness must be sensitively approached. As psychotherapies are considered for particular circumstances in cross-cultural situations, multiple factors must be considered. It cannot be assumed that particular psychotherapies are universally applicable to specific diagnoses.

Immigrant youth is a very diverse population. Cultural realities for immigrant youth may be largely Western or non-Western or combinations from diverse immigration backgrounds and mixing experiences. The cultural realities of the youth and their families will be factors in their experience of psychological problems and their treatment possibilities. As this book explores the challenges of working with this population and treating with psychotherapeutic interventions, the reader must be aware that cultural contexts will underlie the clinical experiences. The possibilities of using psychotherapy cross-culturally must be approached with awareness of the evidence and a critical eye.

References

1. Benjamin Jr LT, editor. A history of psychology: Original sources and contemporary research. 3rd ed. Hoboken, NJ: Wiley-Blackwell; 2009.
2. Goodwin CJ. A history of modern psychology. 2nd ed. Hoboken, NJ: Wiley; 2005.
3. Notterman JM, editor. The evolution of psychology: fifty years of the American psychologist. Washington, DC: American Psychiatric Association; 1997.
4. Reed ES. From soul to mind: the emergence of psychology, from Erasmus Darwin to William James. New Haven, CT: Yale University Press; 1997.
5. Leahey TH. A history of psychology: main currents in psychological thought. 2nd ed. Upper Saddle River, NJ: Prentice-Hall; 1987.
6. Awaad R et al. Obsessional disorders in al-Balkhi's 9th century treatise: sustenance of the body and soul. J Affect Disord. 2015;180:185–9.
7. Arnett JJ. The neglected 95%: Why American psychology needs to be less. Am Psychol. 2008;63:602–4.
8. Diamond J. The world until yesterday. What can we learn from traditional societies? New York, NY: Viking; 2012.
9. Reid PT. The real problem in the study of culture. Am Psychol. 1994;49(6):524–5.
10. McLoyd VC. The impact of economic hardship on black families and children: psychological distress, parenting, and socioemotional development. Child Dev. 1990;61:311–46.
11. Reid PT. Racism and sexism: comparisons and conflicts. In: Katz P, Taylor D, editors. Eliminating racism: profiles in controversy. New York: Plenum Press; 1988. p. 203–21.
12. Brock A. Internationalizing the history of psychology. New York, NY: New York University Press; 2006.
13. Kim U, Yang K, Hwang K, editors. Indigenous and cultural psychology: understanding people in context. New York, NY: Springer Science; 2006.
14. Watters E. Crazy like us: The globalization of the American psyche. New York, NY: Simon and Schuster; 2010.
15. Schwartz JM, Begley S. The mind and the brain: neuroplasticity and the power of mental force. New York, NY: Harper Collins; 2002.
16. Wierzbicka A. Empirical universals of language as a basis for the study of other human universals and as a tool for exploring cross-cultural differences. Ethos. 2005;33(2):256–91.
17. Koenig H. Religion and mental health: what should psychiatrists do? Psychiatr Bull. 2008;32:201–3.
18. Larson DB, Thielman SB, Greenwood MA, et al. Religious context in the DSM-III-R glossary of terms. Am J Psychiatr. 1993;150:1884–5.
19. Ohayon MM. Prevalence of hallucinations and their pathological associations in the general population. Psychiatry Res. 2000;97(2–3):153–64.
20. Verghese A. Spirituality and mental health. Indian J Psychiatry. 2008;50(4):233–7.
21. Dols MW. Majnun: The madman in medieval Islamic society. Oxford: Clarendon; 1992.

22. Jablensky A, Sartorius N, Ernberg G, et al. Schizophrenia: manifestations, incidence and course in different cultures: a world Health Organization ten-country study. Psychol Med Monogr Suppl. 1992;20:1–97.
23. Kulhara P, Chandiramani K. Outcome of schizophrenia in India using various diagnostic systems. Schizophr Res. 1998;1:339–49.
24. Ohaeri JU. Long-term outcome of treated schizophrenia in a Nigerian cohort. Retrospective analysis of 7-year follow-ups. J Nerv Ment Dis. 1993;181:514–6.
25. Thara R. Twenty-year course of schizophrenia: the Madras Longitudinal Study. Can J Psychiatr. 2004;49:564–9.
26. Karno M, Jenkins JH. Cross-cultural issues in the course and treatment of schizophrenia. Psychiatr Clin North Am. 1993;16:339–50.
27. Ribeiro BT. Coherence in psychotic discourse. Oxford: Oxford University Press; 1994.
28. Kleinman A. Rethinking psychiatry: From cultural category to personal experience. New York: The Free Press; 1988.
29. Lewis-Fernandez R. Cultural formulation of psychiatric diagnosis. Case No. 02. Diagnosis and treatment of nervios and ataques in a female Puerto Rican migrant. Cult Med Psychiatry. 1996;20:155–63.
30. Robins LN. Epidemiology: reflections on testing the validity of diagnostic interviews. Arch Gen Psychiatry. 1985;42:918–24.
31. Kirmayer L, Young A, Robbins J. Symptom attribution in cultural perspective. Can J Psychiatr. 1994;39:584–95.
32. Lewis-Fernandez R, Kleinman A. Cultural psychiatry. Theoretical, clinical, and research issues. Psychiatr Clin N Am. 1995;18:433–48.
33. Kleinman A, Kleinman J. Suffering and its professional transformation: toward an ethnography of interpersonal experience. Cult Med Psychiatry. 1991;15:275–301.
34. Simons RC. The resolution of the Latah paradox. J Nerv Ment Dis. 1980;168:195–206.
35. Simons RC. Latah II – problems with a purely symbolic interpretation. J Nerv Ment Dis. 1983;171:168–75.
36. Simons RC. Boo! Culture, experience and the startle reflex. Oxford: Oxford University Press; 1996.
37. Geertz H. Latah in Java: a theoretical paradox. Indonesia. 1968;5:93–104.
38. Kenny MG. Latah, the symbolism of a putative mental disorder. Cult Med Psychiatry. 1978;2:209–31.
39. Kenny MG. Paradox lost: the latah problem revisited. J Nerv Ment Dis. 1983;171:159–67.
40. Colman, A.M. A dictionary of psychology. Oxford: Oxford University Press (2001).
41. Simons, R.C. Introduction to culture-bound syndromes. Psychiatric Times, (2001);18(11). Retrieved February 15, 2007, from http://www.psychiatrictimes.com/p011163.html.
42. Rutter M, Nikapota A. Culture, ethnicity, society and psychopathology. In: Rutter M, Taylor E, editors. Child and adolescent psychiatry. 4. Vol. 16. Oxford: Blackwell Publications; 2002. pp. 277–286.

Index

© Springer International Publishing Switzerland 2016
S.G. Patel, D. Reicherter (eds.), *Psychotherapy for Immigrant Youth*,
DOI 10.1007/978-3-319-24693-2

Printed in the United States
By Bookmasters